"Shannon Algeo inquires deeply into the questions that confront all of us now. Like a guide through a very dense forest, he paves a path and sheds light on where we need to walk. His hand is steady, his words encouraging, and the path he creates always moving in the direction of our spiritual truth."

> —**Marianne Williamson**, author of *A Return to Love* and *A Politics of Love*

"Honest, earnest, brave, and liberating, Shannon's practices and illuminating narratives in *Trust Your Truth* will guide you home to yourself."

> —**Elena Brower**, best-selling author of *Practice You*

"Shannon is a gifted and authentic teacher. He bravely shares the truth of his life lessons and the practices that helped him find clarity, build resilience, and thrive. I highly recommend this book to anyone who seeks to live a fulfilling and abundant life that is aligned with purpose."

> —**Tracee Stanley**, yoga teacher, and author of *Radiant Rest* and *The Empowered Life Self-Inquiry Oracle Deck*

"*Trust Your Truth* is an intimate, well-organized, and thought-provoking spiritual road map that provides embodied tools for healing past trauma, and soulful insights that lead to greater self-confidence. Shannon Algeo's relatable and honest storytelling sets the tone for personal inquiry, and his explanation of the body's energy system (chakras)—and the questions and practices he offers for self-exploration—are intriguing and accessible. *Trust Your Truth* is a meaningful companion for anyone on the path toward healing, awakening, and purpose."

> —**Seane Corn**, yoga teacher; cofounder of Off the Mat, Into the World; and author of *Revolution of the Soul*

"Shannon is pure love. A true healer who is healing himself and sharing his rich wisdom with us. *Trust Your Truth* is a potent and powerful book—a must-read for any spiritual seeker who is looking to go deeper, heal past trauma, and become a beacon of light in this world."

> —**Shaman Durek,** sixth generation shaman; internationally renowned spiritual leader; and author of the best seller, *Spirit Hacking*

"Shannon Algeo is a sage for our times. And his life-changing book, *Trust Your Truth*, is a handbook for living. Vulnerable. Authentic. Uplifting. We are *more* than ready for this message!"

> —**Sheri Salata,** former executive producer for *The Oprah Winfrey Show*; and author of the best-selling memoir, *The Beautiful No*

"Full of depth, knowledge, and wisdom, *Trust Your Truth* honors the fullness of yoga while being accessible no matter where an individual is on their path. Shannon's personal reflections reveal universal truths that invite us to more completely inquire within. He has created a true companion for us all to turn to, grow with, and go with as we navigate incredible external and internal change. This is exactly the book we need right now."

> —**Octavia Raheem,** author of *Gather*, and founder of Starshine & Clay

"*Trust Your Truth* touches your soul and gives the gift of a deeper self-exploration. I am forever touched by Shannon's words, his heart, and the gifts he shares in this highly important book."

> —**Barrett Pall,** professional behavioral change expert, life coach, social media influencer and activist, and host of the *Soul Boners Podcast*

"Reading Shannon's words felt like I was being compassionately and lovingly guided towards the courageous path of coming home to myself. *Trust Your Truth* is the necessary guide to rejoining our soul in its most authentic expression. Thank you, Shannon, for bringing your love and humor to a journey that isn't always joyous."

—**Mark Groves**, human connection specialist; and founder of Create The Love and the emotional wellness app, Mine'd

"This book is a wake-up call pointing us in the direction of our inherent knowing. It is an essential guidebook to navigating the chaos of this moment with skill and grace. Shannon's voice is brave, humble, and provocative in how it makes us question everything we've been taught so that we can remember what we already know. It is an essential call to action to get out of our own way and get engaged in the world."

—**Kerri Kelly**, founder of CTZNWELL, and host of the CTZN *Podcast*

"This book is therapy for the soul. Life can be tough, especially if you've been marginalized in any way. *Trust Your Truth* cuts straight to the core and gives you practical tools you can implement into your life right away to experience massive transformation. Regardless of who you love, what color your skin is, or how much trauma you've been through in your life, Shannon's words will heal you in places you didn't even know were wounded, but that needed your love most. Run (don't walk!) toward this book and read it now."

—**Justin Michael Williams**, author of *Stay Woke*

"Shannon's words are timely. This book is a healing guide to connect us with our higher selves. A must-read."

—**Charles Chen**, founder of www.zzeal.co

"Shannon Algeo takes us on a wonderful and unflinching journey through the 'beauty of a breakdown' in the way that only he can. In order to get to the root of our feelings and perceptions, we have to actually do the work to heal from past trauma. If you're ready to embrace the next level of freedom, *Trust Your Truth* is your guide."

—**Rha Goddess**, founder and CEO of Move The Crowd, and author of *The Calling*

"With this book, Shannon offers the world a brave and heartful blueprint for how to bring more authenticity into the most mundane and exceptional aspects of our lives. Get ready for a journey of growth, compassion, and a whole lot of love!"

—**Anu Gupta**, founder and CEO of BE MORE with Anu

"*Trust Your Truth* is a wonderful book that applies spiritual wisdom to address today's pressing problems and curiosities."

—**Sahara Rose**, best-selling author, and host of the *Highest Self Podcast*

"*Trust Your Truth* is a powerful, practical, and playful guide to a liberated life. Shannon's ability to weave information, education, and his own stories into the book make for an impactful and compelling read. You won't want to put it down, but be sure to do all the exercises!"

—**Lauren Taus, LCSW**, founder of Inbodied Life, psychedelic-assisted therapist, podcaster, and yogi

Trust Your Truth

Heal Self-Doubt,
Awaken to Your Soul's Purpose
& Live Your Badass Life

SHANNON ALGEO

REVEAL PRESS
AN IMPRINT OF NEW HARBINGER PUBLICATIONS

Distributed in Canada by Raincoast Books

Copyright © 2021 by Shannon Algeo
          Reveal Press
          An imprint of New Harbinger Publications, Inc.
          5674 Shattuck Avenue
          Oakland, CA 94609
          www.newharbinger.com

Cover design by Sara Christian; Interior design by Michele Waters-Kermes; Acquired by Elizabeth Hollis Hansen; Edited by Gretel Hakanson

---

Library of Congress Cataloging-in-Publication Data

Names: Algeo, Shannon, author.
Title: Trust your truth : heal self-doubt, awaken to your soul's purpose, and live your
    badass life / Shannon Algeo.
Description: Oakland, CA : New Harbinger Publications, Inc., 2021.
Identifiers: LCCN 2020036754 (print) | LCCN 2020036755 (ebook) |
    ISBN 9781684036998 (trade paperback) | ISBN 9781684037001 (pdf) |
    ISBN 9781684037018 (epub)
Subjects: LCSH: Self-doubt. | Self-confidence. | Mind and body. | Courage.
Classification: LCC BF697.5.S428 A44 2021 (print) | LCC BF697.5.S428 (ebook) |
    DDC 158.1--dc23
LC record available at https://lccn.loc.gov/2020036754
LC ebook record available at https://lccn.loc.gov/2020036755

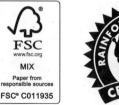 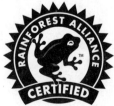

Printed in the United States of America

23   22   21

10 9 8 7 6 5 4 3 2 1   First Printing

For mom and dad, Susan and Michael Algeo, for your infinite love that has shaped me into the person I am. Thank you for encouraging me to be myself and follow my heart. I carry you both with me wherever I go, and I love you with my whole freakin' heart.

♡

Contents

Introduction   1

Chapter 1   You Belong Here. In This Body.   15

Chapter 2   Find Your Own Flow   39

Chapter 3   Power Up Your Soul's Purpose   63

Chapter 4   Let Your Heart Lead   87

Chapter 5   Your Word Is Your Wand   113

Chapter 6   20/20 Vision   133

Chapter 7   Surrender to Source   153

Chapter 8   Be the Whole You. We Need You.   171

Acknowledgments   177

Introduction

"There is something dying in our society and our culture, and there's something dying in us individually. And what is dying, I think, is the willingness to be in denial. And that is extraordinary! It's always been happening, and when it happens in enough of us, in a short enough period of time, at the same time, then you have a tipping point, and the culture begins to shift. And, where people are now is, 'Bring it on. I have to face it. We have to face it.'"

—Rev. angel Kyodo williams, author of *Radical Dharma*, in an interview on "On Being" with Krista Tippett

On my birthday a few years ago, my glass shower door came shattering all over me as I was taking a bath. Little shards of glass cut into my skin as I stood there bleeding into the tub. Happy birthday to me?! Like some kind of fucked-up rite of passage, I had to tiptoe on the glass to get from the tub to the bathroom door. Luckily, I was okay, and instantly, I knew this was a wake-up call. The moment the door shattered, I was angry at a friend who'd canceled our dinner plans. I wasn't trying to break the shower door, but when it got stuck, the intense energy of my frustration informed the way I handled it. As I tried to get it unstuck, it bent in just such a way that it shattered completely. All over me.

Later, I went online and saw that the symbolic significance of glass shattering is "the shattering of illusions." *Oh great.* I did NOT want to see the deeper meaning. *Fuck the company that made this door!*

Fuck my building management for installing a cheap door! Fuck my friend! Fuck the world! Believe me, I went there. I was tempted to take no responsibility. But I also knew there was no power or truth in blame. This heated anger felt all too familiar, so I knew I needed to look underneath the surface of my inner explosion.

When my friend canceled our dinner plans, I got triggered. As I looked underneath the surface of my pain, I could see my old wounded narratives of abandonment and rejection. *I was mad at my friend for "making me" feel this way.* But in truth, my old pals "Unworthiness," "Not Good Enough," and "Not in Control" were coming out to play. I couldn't see past the haze of my woundedness and couldn't even come close to understanding that this had nothing to do with me. The truth was that my friend was feeling so depressed that she couldn't get out of bed.

But my own feelings of brokenness caused the shower to break, and the illusion of woundedness shattered along with the glass. I could suddenly see clearly! I was present and open to receiving this wisdom: *Shannon. You must heal this—this pattern of making someone else's emotional state mean something about your worth. TIME. TO. HEAL. THIS. NOW!!! Your energy is powerful. But YOU are responsible for it. Don't be reckless. Every action you take has an impact. No matter how much you think you can suppress your emotions, you'll either implode or explode because the energy needs somewhere to go. Energy can neither be created nor destroyed. It can only be transferred. Attempting to suppress emotions literally doesn't work. It's time to feel and heal.*

This lesson had come to me many times before. But, to be totally honest, I needed the glass to shatter all over me on my birthday to ensure that I really heard it. But *just in case* I missed it, the Universe came through. The next day, two maintenance guys came to vacuum the glass and clean up, and when they were done, they called me into the bathroom to see their work. I walked toward the shower to peek at the second glass door that still remained intact. I touched it gently and saw that it was stuck. Then, one guy started to fidget with it, and before I could open my mouth to tell him to stop, the other remaining door shattered on top of all three of us. Got it, Universe! I will use shower curtains from here on out, and I will be responsible for my energy! *Message received.*

The beauty of a breakdown is the opportunity it presents for a breakthrough—for you to wake up and become the person you are here to be. As Robert Frost said, "The best way out is always through." We think we're locked in a room with no way out, and then suddenly, we see a doorway we somehow missed. A light at the end of the tunnel. A breath of hope. Breakdown moments are humbling.... We thought our lives were certain, steady, and fixed. And then suddenly, the ground falls out from underneath us. A partner dumps you, a loved one gets sick, the financial markets recede, a global pandemic breaks out, a job is lost, a dream is crushed. Our knees suddenly hit the earth. We are humbled. Grounded. The moments when we break through help us see the patterns that brought us to our knees, build our strength to get back up and step forward onto a new path with deeper gratitude, more wisdom, and a keen sense of what really matters.

These moments of uncertainty and suffering—as painful, confusing, and devastating as they can be—are gateways to profoundly transformative healing and awakening. Listen, I don't want to in any way glamorize or minimize the very real pain of human suffering. *The struggle is real.* We must face the impact of harm done to us and also by us. And at the same time, I know, from my own experience of waking up to my power and reckoning with some hard lessons, that it's so often the moments of deepest despair that lead to the richest insights, healing, and transformation. Some call it "getting hit by a cosmic 2x4."

> The great force
> of life within you
> wants you to wake
> up to the truth.
>
> ♡

Many people miss these lessons though. Even when the lessons seem obvious looking from the outside in, we get caught up in blaming our ex or hating our president or holding onto resentment. We look outside of ourselves for an answer—a scapegoat on whom we can project our discomfort and pain. It's tempting to look for someone else to be the grown-up and take away our problems. But few, if any, spiritual awakenings come from giving our power away to someone else to do the work for us.

You are designed to become conscious of the powerful life-force that you are. The truth within you wants to be seen and felt and deeply known by you. So, when you are living in a fantasy—chasing some dream that you're "supposed to" chase because society says so and unconsciously causing harm to yourself or others by pounding the pavement and trying to fulfill everyone else's expectations—the great force of life that lives within you wants to wake you up to the truth. And, my guess is, because you're reading these words, you're ready. Life has a way of nudging us, of delivering the wake-up call—so we finally hear the voice of our own truth.

At first, life whispers, *"Wake up, sweetheart. It's time."*

But most of us are so busy with emails, scrolling on our phones, and attached to the "certainty" we think we have that we don't hear the whisper. It might come as a gut feeling, thought, or dream. It's hard to miss, but somehow easy to ignore. And so, we remain numb in our busyness and stay the course.

Then, after we've ignored the whispers long enough, life knocks on our door. *"Excuse me. You've got some business to attend to. May I please have your attention?"*

The red flags quadruple in size. You catch your partner in a lie. Migraines beg you for more hydration and rest. You keep changing jobs or moving cities, hoping the next stop will bring you joy and solve all your problems. You feel the same emotional issue come up with your partner that you had with your dad. And your ex. These knocks are harder to ignore. And yet, we can be skillful masters at avoiding our inner work and staying numb.

Then, eventually, the door breaks down. *Yeah, you're gonna need to deal with this. NOW!*

The big thud. The cosmic 2x4. The wake-up call that leaves you feeling naked and vulnerable. It's just you and the whole world open in front of you. A breakup, a job loss, an illness, a global pandemic, a sudden death. *This* wake-up call cannot be ignored and finally awakens the sleeping you.

When you are committed to opening your eyes to the spiritual lessons that life brings you, you open yourself to deeper wisdom and opportunities for healing. Everything is connected, and *nothing* is random. The truth is…sometimes we need the glass door to come shattering down on top of us. Sometimes we need the big loud thud from life. Sometimes it takes death to wake us up to the preciousness of life. But waking up to your truth doesn't always have to involve bloodshed. As we become better at listening for, sensing, and feeling the truth within us, we don't necessarily need to wait for the shit to hit the fan; we can also hear the knocking at the door and even the whisper in our ear.

It's becoming increasingly clear to many. We live in a time where we are being asked to wake up, to become conscious, and to do the inner and outer work to heal ourselves, our communities, and our world. You can choose to be a conscious participant in your awakening, reclaim the power that is your birthright, learn the key lessons that each life experience offers you, and heal the pieces of yourself that have gone unloved for far too long. Or, you can stay asleep at the wheel, give your power away to people and systems outside of you, be a victim to circumstance, and hope that someone sweeps in to save you. I've swung both ways. Each of these choices comes with a cost. If you choose to stay unconscious, you'll close yourself off to the golden treasures of an empowered life—living instead through what seems like a series of random events that are out of your control. If you make the courageous choice to wake up, however, and put in the inner work, you'll open your heart to the possibility of connection to a greater power—and you'll find deep meaning and profound magic in not only the highs of life, but in the mundane and even difficult aspects of your human experience. Trusting your truth requires your presence and willingness. The time is now, and the world is ripe for your truth.

Truth isn't opinionated. It doesn't pick a side. It sees neither good nor bad, right or wrong, up or down, black or white. Truth is *what is.* In her book *The Wisdom of No Escape* (1991), Buddhist teacher Pema Chödrön cites her teacher Chögyam Trungpa Rinpoche as saying, "Buddhism doesn't tell you what is false and what is true, but it encourages you to find out for yourself."

Life doesn't tell you what is false and what is true, but it encourages you to find out for yourself. There is no right or wrong here. No "good" or "bad" way to live your life. This book isn't telling you what is false and what is true, but it's encouraging you to find out for yourself. Your truth is an energy—a quality of awareness—that moves through you. When you desire to wake up, you have less of a tolerance for bullshit and more of a thirst for truth. You actually crave truthfulness instead of fantastical delusions.

Here are some examples of the harmful lies we're sold by society— the myths that we internalize to be "true." The italicized responses to each one are my personal truths. What are yours?

If I buy this expensive bag, my self-worth will increase.

The worth is in ME, not in the bag.

I'm more entertaining to others when I'm drunk. People like me better.

It's not my job to entertain people, and I'm not on this earth to get people to like me. I can be myself.

If I get more likes on this post, I'll feel awesome about myself, and I'll make a real impact.

I am already awesome—independent of this post. If I help one person through this post, that's enough. And, if I'm that one person who gets helped, I am enough.

If she/he/they aren't attracted to me, I'm not physically attractive.

I'm sexy regardless of the fleeting opinions of others.

It's my fault that my boss or partner is abusive. If I could fix what's wrong with me, then I'd be treated with more respect.

I deserve to be treated with the highest quality of respect, love, appreciation NOW. I will not tolerate one more second of mistreatment.

Self-doubt intensifies when we give our power away to people and things outside of us. But your self-worth is always *within you*. This book is an invitation and a guidebook of practices to source your self-worth from the inside out. You can still buy the bag, get drunk, post content on social media, want people to be attracted to you, and navigate complicated relationships, but the difference is that your self-worth will not be tethered to these things. Each time you cut the cord of your self-worth being tied to something outside yourself, you learn to trust yourself just a little bit more.

The gateway to your truth is always through your attention and awareness. So, remember this as you read this book and move through the whole of your life: *your attention is the most valuable resource you have.* It's said, "Where your attention goes, energy flows." Your presence—your life-force—has the ability to dissolve the wildest of delusions. Every time you bring your attention, your awareness, your breath to what's actually happening in this moment now—to what's happening right in front of you—you bring your power back into your body and this moment. When you're stuck playing an old tape of the past or playing out some future outcome, your power is leaking to the past and to the future, and your attention becomes diluted. So, whenever you are wanting to tap into what's true, tap into what's *now*.

As you move through the chapters of this book, you're going to learn practices to trust your truth in each of the seven energy centers of the body—known as the seven chakras (pronounced chock-ras). In the ancient Hindu language Sanskrit, "chakra" means "wheel" or "disk" and is often referred to as a spinning wheel of light. The role of the chakras is to distribute *prana* (life-force energy) through the body. Each chakra has a color, vibration, and truth associated with it. From the lower to the upper body, the chakras are the (1) legs, (2) pelvis, (3) solar plexus, (4) heart, (5) throat, (6) center of the brain, and (7) crown of the head.

Each of these seven energy centers not only exists within a physical location in the body, but also carries symbolic meaning, wisdom, and spiritual lessons for healing. By doing the work in each chapter, you're bringing more conscious awareness to these energy centers within you—and discovering how to live your life according to *your own truth* versus what society or someone else expects from you. You're invited to reckon with any necessary healing that may be required in each energy center—to re-move stuck energy so you can embody your power and trust your truth more fully. The goal is to illuminate your truth on every level of your being—body, mind, heart, and soul—so you can experience your vitality and vibrancy. So that you can practice embodying the lessons of this book, I recorded a Trust Your Truth meditation album, and you can download a guided audio meditation for each chakra/chapter at http://www.trustyour-truthbook.com.

The chapters take you through the chakras sequentially—from the root to the crown—and there's a natural progression to the book. That said, the chakras are a lifelong exploration, so you'll likely relate to them in unique ways as you move through different seasons of your life. Whenever you feel called, you can select a chapter/chakra that resonates with what you're currently going through. Just go to the first page of the chapter, where you'll find a "chakra briefing," read the "Soul Truth," and follow your intuition. While you will, indeed, find lots of information about the chakras in this book, this is less of an encyclopedia of information and more of an experiential, inner investigation for you to discover how *you uniquely relate* to each energy center within you.

The important thing to remember is that *the journey to trust your truth is a practice.* Becoming your True Self is a journey, and you'll have moments where you totally nail it and show up as the true you as well as moments where you default to sleep mode and go back to an old pattern. *That's not only okay; it's often a necessary part of the path.*

Trusting your truth is not about being perfect. It's about showing up to practice. Whenever you align with your truth, you can make choices that bring you closer to your soul's purpose and honor who you really are.

This book is a space to practice being your True Self—the most real, whole, badass YOU that you could ever possibly be. Yes, your True Self is who you're becoming, but it's also important to note that it's who you already are. If you don't yet believe that, my hope is that this book will support you to strengthen your loving relationship with the person reading these words right now.

Here are four essential questions to ask yourself as you navigate this journey:

1. *Who am I becoming?* Each thought you think, word you speak, emotion you express (or suppress), action you make, thing you create, and step you take has an impact. To influence your destiny, become responsible for your reality now. Notice how you're showing up now. Is this your True Self? Your truth asks you to be fully present to who you are in this moment. To not make choices based on who you were in the past or who you think you "should" be, but to instead ground yourself in this moment and be curious about what feels true, loving, and appropriate for you right now.

2. *What would make me proud of myself?* This is one of the most transformative practices I've explored. By identifying what is aligned with your True Self and then doing the things you know will make you proud, you build trust with yourself. You instantly become the person you want to be—and it feels amazing! For example, I know I'll always be proud of myself for doing my morning meditation. So, whenever I meditate in the morning, I feel deep gratitude toward myself because I contributed to my bank account of self-trust. The value of my

self-trust account increases each time I do something to honor my True Self. *Cha-ching!*

3. *What is being activated within me—for the purposes of healing?* The moments when you're triggered can be profound invitations to heal. When you're triggered by something, as difficult as it can be, notice if you can stay open to the information the body is communicating to you. By allowing yourself to fully feel what comes up, you can learn and grow. We'll go much deeper into this in chapter 1 and throughout the book.

4. *How is my healing healing?* Yes, you read that right. How is your personal healing, healing others? When you heal something within yourself, your healing has a ripple effect outward into your relationships and community. Notice this as you do the work in this book. The invitation is to harness your own personal healing to help the world heal because we are all connected. So many of us experience the same inner struggles, face the same demons, and endure human suffering. When we heal, it is our responsibility to be helpers. Sharing is caring.

I'll pose questions (like the ones above) throughout this book. These questions are tools for you to move into deeper self-inquiry, and you may want to journal out your answers. As a helpful tool, you can receive a Trust Your Truth: Journaling Prompt Guide containing all of the journal prompts of this book—organized by chapter. This is a space for you to receive the insights and wisdom that emerge from answering the questions. You can download the guide at http://newharbinger.com/46998 and also benefit from a bonus chapter on gratitude and pivoting.

As I wrote the proposal for this book, I spent a few months living in a small, old one-bedroom apartment in Hudson, New York—a timeshare for artists creating their art. In the hallway that runs from the living room to the kitchen, this quote from *The House on Mango Street* (1984) by activist and poet Sandra Cisneros is plastered in huge red letters on the drywall—from the high ceiling all the way to the floor, "We do this because the world we live in is a house on fire, and the people we love are burning."

We live in a time where there is much less tolerance for bullshit and a real thirst for truth. People are waking up to just how necessary it is that we reckon with our personal and collective pain and trauma. The age of numbing our pain is coming to an end because we're beginning to see how inextricably connected we all are as inhabitants of this planet. We're ready to put a stop to the perpetuation of harm that we unconsciously do to ourselves and each other. The survival of our species actually requires that we wake up now. It's time to heal self-doubt so you can show up for your soul's true purpose and be of badass service to our world. We need you.

On a global level, we see wildfires, pandemics, and melting ice caps as if the Earth herself is crying out for our attention. On a societal level, we see the rise of movements like #MeToo and #BlackLivesMatter—millions of people coming together to collectively demand truth and justice. On personal levels, we see how suicide, addiction, disease, stress, anxiety, and past trauma make it sometimes nearly impossible for us to cope and move forward. And yet, move forward we must.

We are called now to be better stewards of this planet because this is our only home. To be better siblings to each other because we are all one big family—loving, and dysfunctional, and learning. To be better to ourselves because this body is the home base of our soul for this lifetime. As you set out to do this healing work within yourself, may you remember it has a ripple effect beyond your imagination—and has the power to heal the world.

So, before we officially begin our journey together, there are a few things I'd like you to know about the exercises in each chapter:

1. The words, stories, and practices in this book are signposts to point you in the direction of remembering your truth—what you already know to be true deep within you. These words are not the answers, they are gentle invitations for you to go inside yourself and remember the power that lives within YOU. This book may be a guide, but you are the courageous traveler who takes the journey.

2. When doing an exercise, you may notice fear start to bubble up. Fear is normal and can come up in different forms, like resistance, avoidance, overeating, scrolling social media, drugs, alcohol, sex, and the list goes on. When fear arises as you're doing healing work, it is often a sign you are moving toward a tender wound. The invitation is to practice gentleness and compassion with your sweet self. Be kind as you rewind into certain things from your past.

3. Everyone's experience is different and unique. Whenever I offer a meditation or journal exercise, you may want to dive right in, or you may wish to read the whole book and then go back to the exercises. You never "have to" do a practice if it doesn't feel safe or appropriate for you. It's always your choice whether or not you want to engage with the practice. Remember, your healing journey can be whatever it needs to be to best suit you. It's okay to move at your own pace. Little steps are big wins with this type of work.

4. I applaud you for your courage to explore these practices, knowing that some of them may bring up discomfort for you. If you are willing to give a "scary" exercise a try, you may receive great insight. Notice when it feels appropriate to jump right in and just do the work. You got this!

It's time to trust your truth. To deepen your connection to your True Self. To be your own trusted friend and partner on this path of life. Nobody is going to spend as much time with you in this life as YOU, so you might as well learn to be with yourself, love ALL aspects of yourself, and trust your True Self. One of the most courageous journeys is the journey inward. So let's go in, get deep, and explore the vast wisdom, wonder, possibility, and badassery of your own inner world. It's time to heal self-doubt, awaken to your soul's purpose, and live your badass life. Buckle up. Let's go!

CHAPTER 1

You Belong Here. In This Body.

Root Chakra, *Muladhara*

Color: Red

Element: Earth

Body: Immune system, skin, rectum, skeleton, bones

Emotional Impact: Family of origin, sense of belonging, relationship to community, groundedness, and home

Shadow: Fear

Light: Belonging

Soul Truth: *We are all connected to each other.*

Mantra: *Lam* (Bringing the awareness to the legs and feet, repeat "lam"—sounds like mom—out loud or silently eight times before beginning to read this chapter. Sense the energy of groundedness.)

If you're like me, your body hasn't always been a safe place to be. Maybe because of your race, gender, sexual orientation, level of physical ability, religion...the list goes on. Perhaps you currently struggle to feel safe and at home in your body now, or maybe this is something you've struggled with in your past. It's even possible that your struggle to feel safe may be historical and intergenerational—and, through the passage of DNA, the tensions of your ancestors may be alive in your body today. Your brave courage to heal can be the balm that liberates not only your body, but the body of your entire family line. You deserve to find safety and be at home within yourself.

When you first felt unsafe in your body, you likely developed coping mechanisms so you could manufacture a sense of safety and protect yourself. These coping mechanisms now live in the body as habits, defenses, personality traits, and stress levels. While they may have been useful to you in one period of your life (and may even continue to be useful in some moments), ultimately, these defenses become barriers on your path of becoming the true you. In this chapter, we're looking at when you first felt unsafe in your body so you can reckon with the work required to heal. So you can let go of *who you are not* and fully embody *who you are.*

You deserve to live in a world—and in a body—in which you are not just safe, but proud to be yourself. This is a healing process. To heal means to make whole again, retrieving the parts of your lost self and integrating those disowned parts back into the whole of who you are. If there's any part of you that has been disregarded by society, your family, or even yourself, now is the time to cultivate a loving, compassionate, and empowered relationship with yourself and your inner world. It's time to be fully you and feel safe with yourself.

WHAT IS A BODY, ANYWAY?

When people recognize my body, they call it "Shannon." My physical form indicates to them who I am. But at the same time, have you ever had the thought, *I am more than this physical body?*

Isn't there more to you than *just* your physical form? There's also the sound of your voice; the vibe you give off; and your personality, thoughts, desires, sense of belonging, creative potential, and purpose. There's a lot more that goes into making you, *you!*

I remember when I graduated college and moved home for a few months; my family had to put our yellow lab Lucy to sleep because she was so sick. Lucy was a kooky little creature, not big like most labs. She had a "quirky personality" (code for total weirdo) and strong energy. When I was sitting with her on the floor of the veterinarian's office, sadly waiting for Lucy to take her last breath, I felt a powerful sense of sudden peace at the exact moment she left her body. Her energy was contained in her physical form, and then, suddenly, it felt like she was everywhere in the room. I was so keenly aware that the energetic being we called "Lucy" was no longer stuck in her physical dog body. In that single instant, I gained a sense of spiritual knowing that she was everywhere and would forever be with me. Energy can neither be created nor destroyed. It can only be transferred. "You are not your body" made total sense to me in that moment and lives with me to this day.

We *are* more than our bodies. So much more. And yet, our bodies are the channel—the vessel—through which we have this wild, human, and spiritual experience we call life. You are here on this earth—and, for this time, this body is the place you call home. Welcome home.

THE PATH OF BODY-REVERENCE

The reason we start the healing journey by connecting to the body is this: if we don't have a truthful relationship with our body, we struggle to trust ourselves and access our personal truth. Body-reverence is the practice of honoring the physical body—just as it is right now—as the vehicle through which your soul expresses itself in this life.

Body-reverence begins with a deep excavation of all the internalized messages you've received from society that disempower you. For example, body obsession is misperception because when you think you are your body, you mistakenly think your worth is tied to it. The core lies sold to us are "If you look or behave a certain way, you'll be seen, accepted, loved, and given opportunities for survival and success," and "If you don't look or behave a certain way, you are unworthy of being seen, accepted, loved, and given opportunities for survival and success."

Body-reverence is a defiant practice of truth that says: *I'm worthy because I'm here. I am whole, perfect, and complete—just as I am right now, AND I'm continually healing and growing. I deserve to be here.*

Loving your body as a sacred vessel that carries you through this life defies thousands of years of being taught to shame and disconnect from it. Every time you celebrate the breath, mobility, and capacity of your body—despite whatever limitations it may have—you transcend those old narratives and pave a new path forward.

Can you see the body for what it truly is: a temporary temple and the house of the soul—the house *you* live in? It will be yours for as long as you walk this earth. Let's wake up from our collective sleeping state by remembering the wisdom and intelligence that lives within the body.

THE FIVE ENERGY BODIES

Your body may be your home, but it's not the *whole* truth of who you are. Your energy field is bigger and deeper than you can see, feel, and touch. To tap into your truth and let go of the narratives that society places upon you, it's important to understand—and experience—your depth. Yoga Nidra is the "art of transformational sleep" or "enlightened sleep." It's a deep relaxation practice of becoming awake to the areas within yourself where you are sleeping—of becoming conscious of the nonconscious aspects of yourself. Because we live in a society that disproportionately favors the external—the physical, material world—we automatically place more value on physical appearance, money, status, and the stuff our five senses can interact with. We overvalue what's going on *outside of us*, and we undervalue what's going on *inside of us*.

The ancient yogic texts, the Upanishads (pronounced ooo-pahn-eh-shods), teach about the five koshas. In Sanskrit, *kosha* means "house" or "sheath." Each kosha is an energetic layer within you that moves from form (physical) to formless (spiritual/energetic). Think of each layer as the ripple of a wave that's moving from the external world to your internal world and then back again from the inside to the outside. Kamini Desai, author of *Yoga Nidra: The Art of Transformational Sleep* (2017), describes the deepest kosha, the Bliss body, as the vastness of the entire ocean, and the most superficial kosha, the Physical body, as the manifestation of a single wave of the ocean. The single wave is never separate from the ocean from which it emerges, but it is more distinct. Your Physical body is the single wave—the most dense, external expression of who you are. But it's only one sheath—an outward expression of your deeper consciousness, your True Self. When you look in the mirror, you see the wave. When you close your eyes and go inward, you sense the ocean.

Each of the five koshas is an energetic layer that exists between the whole ocean (Source) and the single wave (your Physical body). Moving from the most tangible/seen to the most subtle/unseen, they are:

Ana: Physical body

Prana: Energy body

Mana: Mental body

Vijnana: Wisdom body

Ananda: Bliss body.

The five koshas hold the memories of every experience you've ever had, joy you've ever felt, and trauma you've ever endured. They support you in embodying your full truth because you are becoming aware that your power is more subtle, potent, and deep than you previously knew. Let's explore each.

Anamaya Kosha: Physical Body

Ana means "food," and *Anamaya kosha* is literally the food body. It is the most physical, dense, material, and tangible form that we can touch and hold.

Remember, the five koshas are all inextricably connected to each other. When you solely relate to yourself and build your life around the Physical body, you deny yourself conscious access to your true power. It's as if you owned a house and never realized you could move in, set up some nice furniture and art, ignite a fire in the fireplace, and enjoy your life at home.

Pranamaya Kosha: Energy Body

Pranamaya kosha is the body's capacity to sense and feel sensation. Prana, "life force," is the pulsation of energy throughout your entire system. You can't see or touch sensation, but you can feel and sense it. Can you feel the aliveness in your hands right now? How about your feet? When prana ceases to exist, the physical body becomes lifeless. This was the energy that I sensed leaving Lucy's body when she transitioned. Her physical body was still in the room, but her prana had been lifted.

Manamaya Kosha: Mental Body

The Mental body is the body made of thought—where you take in data and process, label, and categorize information. The Mental body is even subtler than the Physical and Pranic (Energy) bodies. You can't quite put your finger on a thought, but thoughts are energy and have an impact, as they create a ripple effect that influences your words and actions.

Vijnanamaya Kosha: Wisdom Body

The Wisdom body is even closer to the ocean of Source within you. *Vijnana* means "the power of judgment or discernment." The Wisdom body is the higher mind—the means through which you process all of your past experiences, learned information, and intellect so you can make wise choices from a higher-minded state of awareness—from your heart. The Wisdom body learns from past experiences, but it also gleans intuitive insights directly from the Source itself.

This higher knowing connects you to the truth that—at your true essence—you are infinite. Your infinite nature is real, and the false perceptions and limitations you come to believe about yourself are unreal. The Wisdom body allows you to get in touch with your heart and the truth that *all you'll ever need is already alive within you.* Our work throughout this book is a practice in awakening (and remembering) the wisdom and intelligence within your heart.

Anandamaya Kosha: Bliss Body

This is the deepest aspect of who you are—your deepest level of consciousness. If Source is the ocean, then the Bliss body is the subtlest movement of water that begins to initiate the first stages of a wave. It's the *cause* from which all other *effects* emerge. When you come into conscious contact with the Bliss body, you are one with the ocean of Source and experience Oneness. Humans rarely tap into the Bliss body consciously, and most people only experience this bliss *unconsciously* when they sleep.

When you are in a chronic state of tension and stress, it's virtually impossible to consciously access the Bliss body, and yet, it's always present. It constantly stores information through *chitta*, which is like a hard drive that codes and memorizes all our experiences and memories. By developing more conscious awareness of the Bliss body, you can experience transcendent states of deep peace, rest, and Oneness. This is incredibly restorative and healing because you are coming into contact with your true nature. You can consciously access the wisdom files stored in the chitta "hard drive" and begin to heal yourself at the level of cause instead of trying to fix yourself at the level of effect. Would you rather treat the symptoms or heal the cause of a problem?

When I try to treat the symptoms without awareness of the cause of a problem I'm having in my life, the coffee isn't hot enough, I don't like the sound of my yoga teacher's voice, I wish the clients would email me back faster, I want that guy to like me…*I want something on the outside of me to make me feel like I am enough.* The lie that treating the symptoms tells us is, "If this one thing could just be different, I would feel whole again." This is a distraction from going to the Source to heal the cause.

When I access the Bliss body, which is possible through the profound surrender that occurs in the practice of Yoga Nidra, I return home to my enough-ness. I actually *experience* the wholeness that I am erroneously seeking by attempting to control my external world or "get" something from someone outside of me. And! When I let go of the tension and gripping and am able to return home to bliss, an aha moment often occurs: I might realize I need to have a difficult conversation with a loved one that I was deeply avoiding. That my anger at a barista was actually sourced from a desire to be heard by someone I love. *Awareness of the Bliss body helps us access what truly matters.* But, if we stay distracted in our busyness and numbing, we'll keep it surface-level—only engaging in the physical world of tangible stuff we can feel "certain" about. The practice of busyness is a practice of incessant *doing.* The practice of letting go is a practice of *being,* which opens you up to become available to receive the inner wisdom that is already alive within you.

Through enhancing your awareness of these five bodies of energy within you, you can access your deep truth. I recorded a Yoga Nidra meditation for deep relaxation for you to experience the five koshas and surrender into your enough-ness. You can practice at http://www.trustyourtruthbook.com.

ROOT CHAKRA AND THE IMPACT OF TRAUMA

The element associated with the root chakra is earth, and your physical body—your skin, bones, muscles, organs, and cells—make up your earth and allow the space for you to live, be, survive, and thrive. The root chakra is connected to safety, security, belonging, and a sense of inextricable oneness with our families of origin and/or chosen community. On the level of the root chakra, our deepest desire is to feel safe and belong. Our deepest fear is that we don't belong—that we are broken and will be kicked out of the tribe. This core fear of not belonging often occurs to the body as a trauma.

Peter Levine, author of *Waking the Tiger* (1997), defines trauma "as anything that overwhelms your capacity to cope and leaves you feeling helpless, hopeless, or out-of-control and unable to respond." Not all trauma is shock trauma, which is sudden and intense, like a car accident or a school shooting. Some traumas are developmental, which means they happen slowly over time through events like bullying, witnessing fights at home, enduring racism and other forms of marginalization, or receiving constant negative messaging about one's body. Both shock trauma and developmental trauma affect someone's sense of being safe in the world and in their body.

My own early life as a little Shannon in Catholic school significantly influenced my sense of safety, security, and belonging. I was a sensitive, tender, geeky little kid—more effeminate than other boys in my class. Most of my friends were girls, *and* because my name is Shannon, I was constantly targeted and bullied in school from the day I arrived nearly till the day I left. It started with "Shannon's a GIRL's name!!!" from most of the boys. This would escalate to getting pushed around in the bathroom. And by the time I was six years old, I could barely get through the school day without hearing, "You fucking faggot!" or "GAY!" as I walked down the hallway. There was little place for a boy to be sensitive, tender, and unique in this environment. Boys were supposed to be macho, play sports, and hang with the other boys. I wanted to play barbies, sit with my girlfriends, and pluck honeysuckles at recess.

Every day, I was terrified to be at school. And my body felt the impact. I was almost always worried I'd encounter meanness and be ostracized. In the school bathroom, my heart would race and my body would flush with adrenaline, so I avoided going to the bathroom and would do my best to hold it in all day. In sixth grade, when most of my classmates started chatting online, the threats got nastier and more severe. The overarching message I heard was: "You are different. You are wrong. You don't belong." One of my teachers once told my parents in a parent-teacher conference, "Maybe if Shannon was more like the other boys, he wouldn't have so many problems." Being true to myself in the presence of others was often risky—and it always came with a cost.

It's alarming and infuriating how dominant patriarchal culture robs so many little boys of their sensitivity and their tenderness, how we tell boys and girls who they can be based on outdated models of gender "norms." I was constantly told, "Be tough," "Don't be a pansy," and "Man up!" But no matter how hard toxic masculinity tried to squeeze my honeysuckle self into its tight little box, I couldn't fit in.

When you have to defend yourself at such a young age, you quickly learn a thing or two about who you truly are. Don't get me wrong: I wouldn't wish these experiences on any little ones, and no child should have to endure this. *And,* I also see how these experiences pushed me to connect to who I am on the *inside*—regardless of the opinions of others.

Before I could grow from this experience, I needed to reckon with the impact. Remember, trauma is *"Anything that overwhelms your capacity to cope and leaves you feeling helpless, hopeless, or out-of-control and unable to respond."* For ten years, I lived in that state. Little Shannon started to believe these hateful messages he was hearing, so as an adult, I've had to reckon with the *internalized* bullies that still tell me I'm somehow broken, unworthy, and don't belong. These external messages turned into my own internal negative beliefs about myself. Similarly, your earliest, formative life experiences influence your sense of safety and belonging in the world. Based on how safe you felt in your body growing up, patterns and habits began to take root so you could cope with *your* conditions.

The thing about trauma is: If we don't process it, it continues to live in the body, as do the coping mechanisms we develop to keep ourselves safe. As the saying goes, "The issues are in the tissues." When something traumatic happens to us and we feel unsafe to be ourselves, our body reacts by shifting into a sympathetic nervous system response, also known as fight, flight, or freeze. In this state, the body releases the hormones adrenaline and cortisol, and the blood rushes away from the stomach and toward the limbs to prepare the body to either (a) run as fast as it can or (b) fight the damn dragon. The heart is pounding, the skin begins to sweat, and the breathing becomes fast and quick. This is a chemical response to a perceived threat. On a purely physical level, this can lead to lower immune function, trouble with digestion, insufficient quality of sleep, and the list goes on.

The body remembers everything, and Anandamaya kosha, the Bliss body, is where chitta stores information and data about every experience. If you had to endure this type of fight-flight-freeze response as a normal status quo in your early environment as a child, it's likely you developed some coping mechanisms to deal with it. And whether you fought, fled, or froze, the body went into a state of contraction to protect itself from the harm. As I learned from my friend and mentor Seane Corn, internationally renowned yoga teacher and author of *Revolution of the Soul* (2019), contraction without release becomes chronic tension. Tension without release becomes stress. And prolonged stress without release becomes disease. Simply put, dis-ease is a lack of ease in the body. When our bodies are in a state of dis-ease, the answer is not to fight and combat stress with more tension (although that may be your first impulse). We want to create intentional space for release, rest, and ease.

When coping mechanisms become our normal ways of dealing with the world, they can happen so automatically that we don't even question them. Or, if we do question them, they can bring up so much shame because we know we are reacting from woundedness. Either way, we're disconnected from the truth.

We can't stop the world from having an impact and harming us, but we can rise up and heal. We can become who we're meant to become despite these experiences and use them for our growth. This is post-traumatic growth. These are five healing practices to transcend this body trauma—this sense that you don't belong in your body—and to create new ways of being true to yourself:

1. Get to the roots of your core wounds.

2. Expand your capacity to cope (with clarity and compassion).

3. Practice and process healthy discharge and release through movement.

4. Create a brave, safe container for healing from the inside out.

5. Belong to your True Self.

1. Get to the Roots of Your Core Wounds

To create an inner environment where you feel secure in who you are so you can embody your truth, you must courageously dig into the roots of insecurity. It takes both practice *and* courage to go deep and explore the impact of those early-formed memories. The invitation here is to reflect on the experiences that overwhelmed your capacity to cope and left you feeling helpless, hopeless, out-of-control, or unable to respond. Ask yourself and write in your journal:

When did I first feel unsafe in my body? Unsupported? Ostracized? At risk?

Why did I feel like I didn't belong?

What is the story I told about myself and maybe even believed?

What was the impact of "not belonging" on my body?

I'll say this here and now because it needs to be said:

Despite your experiences and any traumas you've endured, remember, you are not damaged or broken. *You are healing.* Your soul work is to heal the root impact of the wound so you can be free from its nonconscious grip on your life. As you go to the roots to heal, you create new possibilities for power and purpose. Because of this work, you get to write new narratives and have new life experiences.

It's important that as you practice bringing the shadow to the light (reckoning with the impact of trauma), you *also* practice bringing the light to the shadows (being gentle with yourself and remembering your capacity to heal and grow). Deep breaths. Be kind.

2. Expand Your Capacity to Cope

The coping mechanisms I developed to protect myself from bullying were useful to me at the time. I'd get defensive when bullied, and I'd express my anger at home (I once punched a windowpane in my childhood bedroom and kicked a big, tall mirror that created a huge crack in the shape of the letter S, which was unfortunate, but secretly, I thought was cool!). I also became obsessed with reading other people's energy to assess whether or not they were a threat.

As an adult, when I feel threatened, this is how these nonconscious patterns play out for me: My body has a fight-flight-fear response to criticism because it perceives any kind of criticism as bullying. I get defensive when receiving almost any kind of feedback as a means to protect myself from the potentially harmful opinions of others. When I prioritize pleasing others and I take on too much responsibility, I can become resentful and frustrated. And, if I'm not being fully conscious and present, I can read someone's energy and morph into the person they want me to be so I stay safe instead of standing in the truth of who I am.

I've come to understand that while I know these experiences of bullying have left an indelible mark on me, I am not broken. I honor the coping mechanisms for how they've shown up to keep me safe. And, I acknowledge how these mechanisms can lock me in a box that is centered around the core trauma of not belonging.

The greatest danger of being told by the outside world that you don't belong is *you might actually believe it.* This is the most common travesty, and this is what we must unravel together. Any part of you that mistakenly believed—or still believes—that you don't belong *is where the work is!* Now is the time to courageously venture into those unhealed spaces and shed the light of belonging.

I invite you to do some self-inquiry and reflection to see the coping mechanisms that you may have formed to ensure you could stay safe and maintain a sense of belonging. Reread your responses to the journaling questions I posed above. Then, ask yourself and journal:

What coping mechanisms did I develop in order to maintain a sense of safety and security?

As you write, let your body answer the question. Oftentimes, we underestimate the wisdom that lives within us—and there's a wellspring of wisdom inside the body. Notice if you are overthinking it and just get your pen onto the page and let your body write the answers. Notice your breath. Even if it makes "no sense" at first, just keep writing. The body has the power to reveal its wisdom if you let it speak. Let your Vijnanamaya kosha, Wisdom body, have the floor, and see what spills out onto the page.

3. Time to Discharge. You've Got to Move It, Move It

Movement is one of the most effective, and essential, methods of discharging old, stuck, historical energy in the body. Movement is medicine. Dancing, twerking, jumping jacks, running, yoga, sweating, hiking…you name it. All of these forms of movement (and others not listed) can be activated as tools for releasing stored tension, stress, and trauma in the body. Move it to lose it! Movement also helps release endorphins, those "feel good" chemicals in the brain.

DANCE

Put on a great tune and start twerking! I'm not even kidding. If you're in a funk or feeling like you have pent-up aggression or tension of any kind, get that booty bouncing! Move it to lose it. When I first started taking dance classes, I was eleven, and I swear I had eleven left feet. Who cares how it looks; get a pulse on how it FEELS. And just fucking dance. The mind might not even understand what the body needs to discharge; the body just needs a release. In our culture, we consume a lot of information through technology, social media, streaming TV, and our busy lives. It's essential to have an outlet for the body to unload everything it's holding onto—most of which we don't even consciously realize is impacting us. Twerk, my love.

YOGA

Yoga means "union" or "to yolk." Through breath and movement, we integrate the body, mind, heart, and soul into Oneness. Yoga has been a transformative healing practice for me to connect to the power and strength of my body. Find a yoga teacher, class, or style you love. There are many styles of yoga out there, so keep searching and keep going until you find a teacher or style that resonates with your body. There's vinyasa, hatha, Iyengar, Jivamukti, Forrest, ashtanga, hot power, slow flow, Accessible Yoga, heck, there's even goat yoga. Find what strikes your fancy. *And pro tip*: Develop *your* yoga practice and it will become a part of your life practice. Now, if I go a week without doing yoga, my body craves it. My yoga practice helps me feel whole, and now my body knows what whole feels like. This reference point of wholeness is stored in the chitta of my Bliss body, and my Wisdom body communicates when it's time to practice yoga through a message that sounds something like, "Girl, it's time for you to do some yoga. Get on your mat!"

SWEAT IT OUT

High-intensity interval training (HIIT) workouts, cardio kick-boxing, spinning, or any kind of intense strength training has been an essential practice for me to process frustration, anger, and rage as well as build physical strength. Cardiovascular workouts really get your heart pumping and are good for your lymphatic system, which supports your immune health. Unlike the circulatory system, which pumps on its own, the lymphatic system requires movement to release fluid. Cardio and strength training are great ways to shift your state from a lower, more lethargic vibe to a higher, more lively vibe. This type of movement almost always gives me that feeling of, *"YES! I AM A TOTAL BADASS!"* (even when the workout is totally kicking my ass). If vigorous movement is inaccessible or undesirable for you, you may consider releasing toxins by sweating it out in a dry sauna or steam room or by laying out in the sun (don't forget your SPF!)

HIKE OR NATURE WALK

Whether it's a barefoot walk in your backyard, a beautiful hike, or just a walk outside, being in the elements of nature is healing and purifying. Receiving the negative ions from the surrounding plants and trees, getting fresh air, and moving the body through space is so simple, yet so profound. Get out of the house and practice receiving the elements from your surrounding space.

CHECK IN WITH YOUR INTENTION

Whatever movement you choose to practice, notice the *energy behind the movement*. What's the intention? Sometimes you can put yourself through a hard, exhausting strength training workout to build up your confidence, and other times you can put yourself through the same workout as a means of self-punishment. Cultivating an empowering relationship with your body is not a one-size-fits-all fix. When you reach into the movement medicine cabinet, check in with what practice you are choosing and why.

Ask yourself:

How is this practice a way for me to love, empower, and be kind to myself?

How is this practice an act of honoring my True Self?

For a Movement Medicine Practice fusing some fun dance, yoga, and a touch of high intensity training led by me, go to http://www.trustyourtruthbook.com.

4. Create a Brave, Safe Container

In an excerpt from "Invitation to Brave Space," Micky ScottsBey Jones says,

"Together we will create brave space
Because there is no such thing as a 'safe space'
We exist in the real world.
We all carry scars and we have all caused wounds."

We can't guarantee a safe space in this very real world. Race, gender, level of physical ability, sexual orientation, socioeconomic status, access to resources, and health all influence an individual's ability to feel safe in their body. That said, we *can* do our very best to heal our inner space and create an internal environment of safe space within. As each of us bravely sets forth to heal the impact of external harm and create a safe space within, we increase our ability to create a safer, more compassionate, healed, and harmonious external space.

One of the bravest journeys we can take is the journey inward. It's radical to go inward in a culture and society that wants you to conform to external standards for its benefit. Creating a safe space inside yourself through deep relaxation, meditation, and Yoga Nidra is incredibly brave because you are sending a message to your nervous system that it's safe to rest. These practices send a message to your True Self and the entire Universe that YOU are a safe space. We can't control how others show up. But we can control how we show up for ourselves.

When the nervous system shifts into the parasympathetic state, the body is able to "rest and digest." In this state, the body can heal and restore, and your True Self can emerge. Plus, one of the most effective ways to combat disease caused by physical, mental, or emotional stress is to foster a space of ease and rest in the body. Here are some practices you can do to create a safe container for yourself to ground, breathe, and heal.

One of the bravest
journeys is the
journey inward.

♥

PRACTICE GROUNDING

This is so subtle and simple that we don't even think about it because it requires *less doing* and *more being.* Grounding is the practice of becoming aware of the earth—the ground—underneath the body. You can do this seated, feeling the chair or cushion beneath your seat. Or you can do this standing, feeling the texture and support of the ground underneath each foot. You can also do this lying down, feeling the ground holding and cradling you. In whatever position your body is in now, can you become aware of where your body touches the ground and where the ground touches your body? The earth is what creates the container and the space for you to exist and be here. Can you feel how the ground holds you up and allows you to be here? Can you rest into that support just a little bit more?

PRACTICE BREATHING

Now, as you're feeling the ground, can you become aware of the body breathing? As the body breathes in, feel the ground rise up to support and hold the body. As the body breathes out, feel the body release its weight into the earth even more. As the body breathes in, feel the body receiving the ground. As the body breathes out, feel the ground receiving the body. As you read these words, can you notice the body's capacity to breathe on your behalf—without you having to "do" the breathing?

PRACTICE HEALING ENERGY

In whatever way makes sense for you, imagine a warm, healing, light energy. Imagine drawing three rings of golden healing light around the body to create a cocoon of healing light to surround the physical body. One golden ring of light to protect and support the Physical and Energy bodies. One golden ring of light to protect and support the Mental body. And one golden ring of light to protect and support the Wisdom and Bliss bodies. Imagine your entire body being held in a golden cocoon of warm, healing light energy that completely surrounds, supports, and protects you. Take a few moments to pause, feel, and sense this energy holding you. You can invite this image of golden light to surround the body whenever you like as a means to support you in creating a safe container within yourself.

5. Belong to Your True Self

When you feel like you can't be yourself—that you need to show up and be who someone else wants you to be—you run the risk of becoming someone you are not in order to be safe. I invite you to ask yourself this question and then write the response in your journal.

What is a specific example of when I learned "how to be" and "how not to be" in order to belong and be safe?

This is the origin of self-betrayal—where we first began to lose connection with our truest selves. This is where we began to internalize the narratives: "It's not okay to be the real me." "Real me doesn't belong here." "Hide my truth."

Self-betrayal doesn't happen because we want it to or because we're doing anything "wrong." Self-betrayal happens because we want to stay safe...we want to stay part of the tribe...we want to fit in. We do it for survival. And just like all coping mechanisms, it once served a purpose. But it does not serve the full expression of your soul. It does not serve your truth. And so now, as you tend to the inner child who may be afraid of stepping out in this new way, you must also be the "adult in the room" who says to your inner child, "Okay, sweetie. This 'comfort zone' ain't working anymore. It's time to be brave. I can't promise you won't get hurt, but I can promise that now is the time to be you—and the liberation that comes from being your True Self...it's the best in the world."

In her book *The Gifts of Imperfection* (2010), behavioral psychologist and vulnerability researcher Dr. Brené Brown writes, "Fitting in is about assessing a situation and becoming who you need to be to be accepted. Belonging, on the other hand, doesn't require us to change who we are; it requires us to be who we are."

Woof. That lands every time I read it. *Belonging requires us to be who we are.* The costs of fitting in—and not belonging—are high. If we're always changing in order to be "accepted," we'll never be accepted because the person others will be "accepting" won't be the true us!

When we change who we are to fit in, we:

- Desperately seek validation from others

- Feel like we're never enough

- Don't believe people when they compliment us

- Distrust others (and ourselves)

- Are confused about our purpose

- Attempt to scratch an itch with no relief

- Crave acceptance but rarely feel it

- Believe we're not deserving of the success or accolades we receive (imposter syndrome).

But, hey! Belonging is risky too. It means you might not fit in. At least with fitting in, you can kinda fake your way into "looking like" you belong. Belonging takes courage. It means you are willing to stand up and say, "*You may not accept me, but I'm still gonna BE me. You may not get my style, humor, or truth, but I'm going to stand in it anyway. I'm showing up for myself—even if you don't. I trust I'll always belong to myself, and I'll eventually attract like-minded and like-hearted people who see me for who I truly am. Being my True Self is my one true aim.*"

The benefits of belonging are we:

- Accept ourselves wholeheartedly

- Believe people when they love us

- Measure success based on how true we can be to ourselves

- Can be alone and enjoy our own company

- Don't overvalue the opinions of strangers on the internet (and in real life)

- Honor our feelings and trust ourselves.

In order to be true to ourselves, we must have the courage *to be* ourselves. It's by no means a perfect process. I, sometimes, catch myself selling out on my truth to "fit in." It's a practice, and just like anything, the more you practice, the more skilled you become at what you are practicing. Your continuation through the work of this book will strengthen your practice of *belonging to yourself.* This is the path to honoring and loving yourself. And standing in your truth—no matter what. What's one brave thing you can do right now to let your whole body and nervous system know that you belong to yourself?

In order to be true to ourselves, we must have the courage to be ourselves.

♡

CHAPTER 2

Find Your Own Flow

Sacral Chakra, *Svadhisthana*

Color: Orange

Element: Water

Body: Below the navel; hips, pelvis, sex organs, lower digestive organs

Emotional Impact: Creativity, relationship to father and mother, sense of security, money, masculine and feminine energy

Shadow: Guilt

Light: Flow

Soul Truth: *In the eyes of you, I see myself.*

Mantra: *Vam* (Bringing the awareness to the pelvis, repeat "vam"—sounds like mom—out loud or silently eight times before beginning to read this chapter. Sense the energy of fluidity.)

On the journey to trusting your truth, it's essential to look at your relationships with others because relationships give you deep insights into the quality of your relationship with *yourself*.

For so many of us, we're taught to please others, put others' needs before our own, and edit ourselves to conform to someone else's expectations. But here's the deal: You can't *truly* and fully show up for others unless you show up and be true to yourself. You can't *truly* give someone the gift of your love if you are unwilling to receive that love from others—and give it to yourself.

Relationships are the practice ground and the playing field where you rub up against all your bullshit so you can become the highest version of yourself. Just as it takes pressure and extreme heat to form a diamond, the key lessons of our relationships are often revealed to us through pressure and heat. Sometimes relationships are fun, exhilarating, joyful, and a walk in the park. Other times, they're gnarly, painful, traumatizing, and devastating. Either way, relationships are doorways to self-discovery and healing. As we move into the work of looking at the lessons you have learned—and are learning—from past and current relationships, keep this spiritual perspective in mind: see each person you meet as an angel on your path, a messenger, here to reflect back your own power, potential, and inner truth.

The second chakra leads us to find expression and flow in our creative pursuits, relationships, and sexuality. When the second chakra is in balance, you express yourself creatively, you create healthy boundaries between yourself and others, and you have an empowered relationship with your sexuality. When the second chakra is out of balance, your creativity might feel either stagnant/stuck or hyperactive/neurotic, you'll find little to no boundaries in your relationships, and your sexuality might be either nonexistent or obsessive.

The element of the second chakra is water, and *you* are mostly water! According to H. H. Mitchell, in the *Journal of Biological Chemistry* (volume 158, 1945), the brain and heart are composed of

73 percent water, the lungs are about 83 percent water, and the entire human adult body is made of up to 60 percent water. Stay hydrated because you are designed to flow! Fluidity is a part of your true nature.

Whereas the first chakra is about belonging and oneness, the second chakra is about duality and connection to others. If the first chakra is about "we," the second chakra is about "you and me." You can use your creative, second chakra energy in an infinite number of ways: to paint, build bridges, design cities, discover new ways of recycling, reinvent yourself, make babies, eradicate racism, and the list goes on…literally forever. Relationships help show you what you're made of so you can see yourself more clearly, find your flow, and create what *you* are meant to create.

THE DOORWAY OF DUALITY

Oftentimes, you find your truth by, first, living the lie. You find a healthier relationship with yourself through an unhealthy relationship that develops in your life. You experience and appreciate the peak of success and happiness because you know the days of failure and sadness. One of the most surefire ways to find your center is to explore the polar extremes. Just like in swimming, the further you reach, stretch, and kick the water away from the body, the stronger your core becomes. You have to travel to your edges—those experiences in life where you realize, "OH! This is NOT what I want!" in order to know what you really *do* want. You realize, "OH! This is NOT who I am!" in order to discover who you *really* are. There's no north pole without the south pole. No night sky without the existence of the sun. The polar extremes help you learn how to find your true center.

Let this truth be a big old, sloppy permission slip to fuck up and make mistakes. Finding your truth and learning to honor yourself is not about being perfect and getting it right all the time. In fact, it's about taking the lessons learned from chapter 1 about creating a brave and safe space and then bravely going out and making a mess. I'm not saying be reckless in your life, but I *am* saying you don't need to be perfect. Within the duality of perfectionism versus recklessness, can you find your true authentic center by exploring both? If you're a perfectionist, go make a mess!!! If you're a chaotic clutter monster, schedule a cleanup!!! There's wisdom in the center. And through your courage to explore the duality, you gain context, understanding, perspective, and strength. This is how you find your truth.

Let's look at two of the most influential dualities that exist and how they show up to support you in finding the truth of who you are.

Shadow and Light

We all have shadow and light aspects of ourselves. The nonconscious, unseen aspects of yourself are your shadow. This is what you are *not* aware of. The conscious, seen aspects are your light. This is what you *are* aware of. Our shadow is the part of our humanity that is hard to look at: the fear, guilt, shame, grief, rage, lies, delusions, and cynicism. You know, the fun stuff! ;) The light is the part we tend to prefer: the belonging, flow, confidence, power, love, happiness, and hope. By denying the existence of our shadow, we guarantee its nonconscious stronghold over our behavior, thoughts, and lives. Anytime we deny an aspect of who we are, we *become* the very thing we are running from.

By learning to consciously work with the shadow, we become able to love ourselves completely without denying *any aspect* of who we are. In order to embrace the power of our light, we must be willing to embrace our shadow selves. Truth requires that we integrate both.

Masculine and Feminine

Masculine and feminine energy is more energetically nuanced than "male sex" or "female sex." Gender norms have taught men that it's more appropriate to be masculine and women that it's more appropriate to be feminine. But masculine and feminine energy transcends the "rules" about gender norms because these are energies of the Universe that come together within each of us to create a unique concoction of fluidity and expression.

Feminine energy is the energy of the Divine Mother—spacious, being, moon. Without Mother Earth, there would be no space for life to exist. This energy is healing, nourishing, nurturing, fierce, wild, and holds space for all life.

Masculine energy is the energy of the Divine Father—creation, doing, sun. Father Sky is the fiery purpose that inspires movement, and without it, there would be no motivating impulse to act or force necessary to create. This energy is inspiring, protective, warm, loving, creative, motivated, and directed.

Feminine energy creates the space and welcomes attraction. Masculine energy fills the space and inspires action. When you reclaim and integrate both divine energies into your own body and being in a way that is empowering, enlivening, and authentic to you, your unique creative expression becomes palpable, unstoppable, and alive with truth.

RELATIONSHIPS ARE DIVINE ASSIGNMENTS

The metaphysical, psycho-spiritual text *A Course in Miracles* (2008) refers to anything that comes into our lives to help us heal and remember that, at our essence, we are love, as a "learning device." This most definitely includes relationships. Relationships are the curriculum through which your soul learns the specific lessons it's here to learn so you can heal from past harm and pave a new pathway forward. Every relationship is a divine assignment, delivered to help you see yourself more clearly so you can walk the path of your life with more compassion and truth.

Relationships help bring the shadow to the light; they reveal all of the unhealed spaces within you so you can see them more clearly. Relationships are our greatest teachers because they show us where we've disowned ourselves, where we're codependent, where we tolerate mistreatment, and where we need to stand up for ourselves. Relationships also challenge us to set boundaries, communicate our needs, see where we're disempowered, and fully claim our creative potential. They show us what it feels like to be loved, the benefits of being supported by another, and what it's like to be seen and supported. The more we learn to see one another as mirror reflections of ourselves, the more we can honor each other as soul siblings, as family on this path of life.

Relationships can send us skyrocketing into outer space—powered by the fire of life itself—*and* they can send us deep into a ditch of depression and despair. But, the truth is, we couldn't survive without relationships. Heck, we couldn't even exist without them. There would be no gas in our cars, no water pumping into our homes, no carpools, no public transportation, no money in our bank accounts, no sex in our beds, and no food on our tables. It's through working together that we're able to survive. And, relationships can *also* teach you how to thrive—they can support you to become your highest self.

From a spiritual perspective, every person who you come into contact with—no matter how seemingly insignificant or meaningful—is you. When you're head over heels in love with someone, and your beloved is smiling, flirting, and loving you up, your partner is helping you experience the love within your own heart. You like this experience of yourself.

And yet, when that same person speaks to you in a condescending tone that reminds you of the way your father or mother or ex (or fill in the blank) always spoke to you, and you flare up in a fit of rage, your partner is activating your shadow—showing you a space within yourself that requires empowerment and healing. This is not to say it is *your fault* if your partner is speaking to you in a condescending or demeaning tone. But *your internal reaction* gives you direct insight into your healing curriculum. This is exactly what this relationship was designed to bring up...the wound bubbles right up to the surface of your consciousness and comes into the light for healing. This is your soul work, and if you accept the challenge, stay conscious, and are open to the lesson, transformation is inevitable.

KEY RELATIONSHIP LESSONS

Based on our early relationships with our parents or the people who raised us, we were given "templates" for relationships. A template is what was modeled to us; it's what we grew up in and around, the environment we were steeped in, and the dynamics and energetic patterns that were so ingrained as "normal" that we never really questioned them when we were young—even if they might have been really fucked up!

No template is purely good or bad, healthy or toxic. All aspects of relationships have both shadow and light. That said, all of us were given some templates that need to be questioned, reckoned with, and rewritten. Remember, your templates are stored deep in the chitta hard drive in your Anandamaya kosha, the Bliss body. To rewrite the foundational programming of your hard drive, it takes (1) consistent practice and (2) desire. Because your relationships allow you to see what needs reprogramming, they are your most powerful field of practice. If you don't consciously create a new template, the old template will just replay itself out, which is why so many people find themselves in intimate relationships that mirror their old templates.

"I married my father" or "I married my mother" is a thing for a reason.

Take a moment to reflect upon a common problem or issue that keeps coming up in your relationships. Then in your journal, answer this question:

What painful relationship dynamic is repeating itself, leaving me exhausted and frustrated every time?

If there's a relationship dynamic that is continually showing up again and again, with partners, friends, family, coworkers, or any relationship in your life, an old template is revealing itself to you. There's a saying, "If it's hysterical, it's historical." That which triggers you also reveals to you the pathway toward healing. Identifying the old template is the first step before you can rewrite a new one. This step is essential for you to bring old shadow patterns to the light so you can consciously create relationships that are in alignment with your True Self.

When I was growing up, my mom struggled with unprocessed sexual abuse. Through periods of depression, car accidents, and a diagnosis of multiple sclerosis, my mom struggled to process her own childhood trauma and be emotionally present for me at the same time. My dad hustled as a prosecutor, a law professor, and a judge to provide for our family by working long days and teaching most weeknights. In so many ways, my parents created an incredible and loving home for my younger brother, sister, and me, and they always did their best to make sure we knew how much they loved us. And, they are humans who had their own unprocessed traumas—and they weren't given tools to healthily release and process their experiences and emotions.

My dad's father was born in Ireland, never graduated eighth grade, and was a tough disciplinarian—most of my dad's older siblings got "the belt," but he was spared, as the youngest. Like most boys in his generation (and mine), my dad wasn't taught how to handle shadow emotions: the shame, guilt, fear, grief, and rage. Emotions were to be shoveled away. On top of that, he was drafted and fought in the Vietnam War. My dad's way of handling his anxiety and overwhelm was to take the edge off with a few martinis when he got home from work. My mom grew up in a military family that constantly moved around the world, and her sexual abuse was never dealt with by her family. My mom's way of handling her pain was to hide away in her room, protecting herself from the harshness of the world. For years, my parents' relationship was like a hot potato about to explode at any moment. They would pass around the hot potato of pain, hoping the emotional responsibility would land in someone else's lap and the pain would go away.

In order to brace myself and protect myself from the intensity at home, I learned the skill of sensing and feeling my parents' emotions from a mile away. I'd walk on eggshells to keep from waking the sleeping dragon, and I learned to shapeshift and modify my True Self to adjust to my parents' emotional states. As I got older and fed up with the same old patterns playing out, I wanted to call out the bullshit. I could see the miscommunication, the dysfunction, the harm, and the toxicity. I could smell it in the room, feel it in my body, and hear it in their voices.

I made it my sole mission to clean up shop at my house. I would call my parents on their shit; I'd act out, yell, cry, kick mirrors, and punch windows; and I would tell each of them what the other was telling me in "secrecy" hoping they would actually communicate with—and understand—each other. I was obsessed with fixing. I wanted my parents to see what I saw so they could fix it. At the time, I thought that was my job...there was no other option. After years of healing and reckoning, I now see that I felt incredibly out-of-control and wanted to fix their relationship so I could feel safe.

The essence of my old template was, *I need to fix other people so I can feel safe. I am responsible for other people's emotional states. If people I love aren't okay, I am not okay.* Because of the template I unconsciously developed in my early home environment, my ability to feel at peace with myself as an adult became contingent on the people around me being "okay" and at peace. When there was chaos, I would panic, my nervous system would become dysregulated, and I'd obsessively try to control and manipulate my environment and the people in it. I'd morph into the "fixer." I've had to become conscious of and reckon with this pattern because when I fall asleep at the wheel, it automatically repeats itself in my closest relationships with friends, family, and romantic partners.

As exhausting and inconvenient as it has sometimes been for me as an adult to pick up the pieces of the emotional volatility that became my template for relationships, I'm able to see how this trauma carries with it both shadow and light. Because of the high level of sensitivity I developed to be attuned to my parents' emotions and because of my desire to find hope and solutions in the darkest of moments, this is largely why I have a deep calling and ability to help people heal. There is both shadow *and* light in all aspects of the human experience, and in order to see the truth, I must acknowledge both.

Let's look at the key relationship lessons that may be trying to reveal an old template to you right now. As you identify your old template, be cautious if you hear the voice of shame telling you, "You are so fucked up for being this way." That's just an old narrative playing itself out on repeat. This isn't the truth of *who you are.* You are the courageous being who is witnessing these patterns. Your awareness is like a fire that can burn away the old template, and your desire to be your True Self is what allows you to pave new pathways for healing.

Old templates don't just live in our minds; they live in our bodies. After you've identified the painful relationship dynamic that keeps repeating itself, let's go a little deeper. In your journal, answer these questions for inner exploration and self-inquiry:

Review your answer to the previous question. Is there a familiar trigger—a sensation in your body—that lies underneath this repeated dynamic? If so, what does the trigger feel like in your body when this issue comes up?

Where do you feel it? What sensations do you feel?

Imagine wrapping yourself in compassion. Take a deep breath.

What information, or "lesson" for healing, does this familiar trigger have for you?

Let yourself free-write and see what comes up. You may be able to do this work right now, or it may be helpful to do this self-inquiry the next time a relationship trigger emerges. If nothing is showing up for you right now, I invite you to flag this page and come back to these questions when the moment presents itself.

Repeated patterns in our lives (and sensations in our body) help us to see where deeper healing work is required. As an example, when I first moved to Los Angeles, I was going through a tough period with my boyfriend at the time. While I wanted to think that my anger was just circumstantial and specific to him, I knew that when my sister also gave me feedback about my anger, this *really was* something I needed to work on. The sensation in my body felt the same in both relationship triggers. It was frustrating to have the same internal issue coming up in both relationships, but I was grateful for the clarity because it affirmed that this was, indeed, my healing curriculum and something I needed to look at more closely within myself.

In your journal, take a look at the relationship dynamic that you've written—the repeated pattern that keeps showing up for you.

1. *Identify the theme. What is the core-essence of this lesson for you? (For me, my anger toward my ex-boyfriend and my sister was rooted in a need to control other people's emotions and behavior so I could feel safe.)*

2. *How does it feel to identify and name this pattern?*

3. *Trace this feeling back to its point of origin—the earliest you can remember. When did you first feel this way? (This doesn't have to be exact. Just do the best you can.)*

4. *Breathe into how the body feels and imagine developing a wider space of compassion for your younger self.*

5. *Write the "essence of your old template" down as one sentence.*

6. *How has the old template benefited you? What are the strengths you gained from having gone through this experience?*

7. *What is the painful belief you walked away with that is still lingering here today, that you want to heal?*

Isn't this fun?! On behalf of humanity, thank you for doing this work. Your healing starts, but does not stop, with you. The impact of this ripples into your relationships with your loved ones and into your community and, on some level, affects the healing of the whole world. If you want to end a pattern of intergenerational trauma, *you* are the one you've been waiting for. You are the one who's got to say, "The buck stops here." It takes courage to sit through the discomfort of this stuff, but let me tell you, from my experience, it is far better than the pain of repeating old patterns. As the gifted astrologer Chani Nicholas, author of *You Were Born for This*, says, "What you heal in yourself, you heal for your entire family line." This is big work…bigger than you. And yet, *you* are the one who says, "It's time."

My parents have grown so much throughout the years. They often joke now that their marriage was "sometimes *The Love Boat*, sometimes the *Titanic*." I'm lucky to have gone to therapy with every member of my family—and we've even all gone together! Those sessions can be brutal, but the feeling of freedom afterward is priceless. It's been so important for me to reckon with the impact of these patterns because the reckoning has allowed me to get free, let go, forgive, and create a *new* relationship with both my parents and myself. We heal so we can get free.

Soon, you'll be invited to write and create a new template. But first, let the old template simmer while we take a look into some of the most common issues that hinder relationships from being intimate, authentic, empowered, and real. Boundaries, codependency, and sex! Oh my! Call me Fraulein Maria from *The Sound of Music* because these are a few of my favorite things.

Boundaries

"Walls keep everybody out. Boundaries show people where the door is."

— Mark Groves, expert relationship coach and founder of Create the Love

Boundaries help the people you love access the room of your heart. They teach people how you like to be loved. If you put up a wall, hide your True Self, and mask your vulnerability, people won't know how to access you. As a result, you may end up feeling lonely and craving authentic connection. Putting up a wall is often a coping mechanism to help you feel safe. But boundaries show people where the door is.

> Boundaries help the
> people you love access
> the room of your heart.
> They teach people how
> you like to be loved.
>
> ♡

An example of a wall—everybody out! *People suck. I'm not even going to think about communicating what I "want" because everyone ends up hurting me.*

Can you feel the wall? Connection isn't possible here.

An example of a boundary—here's where the door is! *Hey, I'd feel more open to deepening this connection emotionally if we are both on the same page about our relationship desires. Can we have a conversation about this? If we want different things, I may want to move forward with dating other people. Regardless, my true intention is to communicate and get on the same page so we can respect and honor each other through this process.*

Can you see where the door is?

Here's why boundaries are so awesome: You actually get to design the rules of your game, and you make it possible for everyone to win— both you and your loved ones. You teach others—and simultaneously learn for yourself—how to gain access to the most precious gift you have: your True Self.

Our deepest fear about boundaries is that if we set them, we'll lose relationships. As Melody Beattie says in her book *Codependent No More* (1986), "We're so careful to see that no one gets hurt. No one, that is, but ourselves." By remaining boundaryless, we end up betraying and dishonoring ourselves, which just creates a mess for everyone involved. Most of us suck at—excuse me, are *unskilled at*—boundaries because we're just not aware that we have the option of setting them. If you are a "people-pleaser," setting boundaries might be kinda scary. I was definitely fearful when I started. For most of my life, I didn't realize that boundaries were an option. I felt awkward and was afraid to be seen as "needy." The first couple of times I set boundaries, I thought, *Are you telling me I can actually assert my needs, wants, desires, preferences, dislikes, and requests in this relationship? I can actually communicate what I need and then have that desire witnessed, heard, acknowledged…and maybe even MET!? Holy shit!*

Because I had mastered the skill of "reading the room" and morphing into the person I needed to be to instantaneously please everyone in it (not possible, by the way), I had no boundaries for most of my life. My old template told me, *If you just give everything you have away, you'll be loved! If you have needs, they'll walk out on you.* And while that may have worked to get me to "fit in" in certain environments, it could never lead to true belonging. Because I wasn't being the real me with people.

Boundaries mean you get to say no and honor yourself. If you don't think you have a choice about what you *do not want* in your life, you'll default to choices rooted in fear in order to fit in. As you set boundaries that honor your True Self, you start to thrive. So, if you have struggled with owning your ability to assert your needs in relationships and set healthy boundaries, I am here to tell you: *you get to become a boundaries badass.*

These are some of the fears that may arise when you first start to even *think* about setting boundaries:

- "I'm going to hurt their feelings and come across harsh or unkind."

- "This will cause a fight."

- "They might not like me anymore."

- "I'll end up all alone."

- "This relationship might end."

- "_____."

Take a moment to pause and reflect on your own fears about setting boundaries. Do any other fears come to mind for you? In your journal:

What are your reasons for not setting boundaries?

Identify where in your life you know—deep down—you need to set a boundary.

In what ways would setting this boundary benefit your physical, mental, emotional, and spiritual well-being?

Who might you need to have a conversation with to communicate your new boundary?

Now, let's take a moment to look at the most common fears that come up.

#1: *I'm going to hurt their feelings and come across harsh, or unkind.* Let's be clear. If someone's feelings are "hurt" by your boundary, you're not the one "hurting" them. They may have some emotional reaction or response to you setting a boundary, but *you* are not responsible for other people's feelings. That's outside your jurisdiction of responsibility. You are responsible for you!

My sister Molly has been the boundaries pioneer in my family. At first, her boundary-setting made me feel sad, upset, abandoned, and confused because I was not accustomed to her claiming her right to set boundaries. Rather quickly, though, as I accepted and embraced the space she was claiming for herself, I realized, *OMG. If she gets set boundaries, that means I get to, too!* When you set healthy boundaries for yourself in your life, you give everyone else in your life permission to do the same.

#2: *I might cause a fight.* The people who get the most upset when you set boundaries are the ones who benefited the most from you having none. It's important to remember and know for yourself *why* you are setting this boundary and how necessary it is for you to stand up for yourself and claim your physical, mental, and emotional space. Setting boundaries is not always easy, but whenever you make the choice to advocate for your True Self, you actually create a new template—a new way of being in relationships. *This is healing in action.* If a fight happens, give yourself permission to step away and let the other person be with their emotions, and you with yours.

#3: *They might not like me anymore.* The most important measure for success is that *you* like you! They might not like you anymore. But if *you* don't like and aren't true to yourself, whose life are you living? Trust that your truth will attract people into your life who see you for your brilliance, your radiance, and your badassery. Your truth will also repulse some people and send them in the other direction. This is called divine protection.

#4: *I'll end up all alone.* You may feel lonely (and that's okay), but you are never alone. Feeling lonely can be a powerful doorway to connect inward and develop your relationship with yourself. We tend to think of being alone as a bad thing, but aloneness is really spaciousness. A friend once explained to me that when we are alone, we can connect to the truth that we are *all one.* Aloneness is the time and space in which you can remember that you are connected to the *all Oneness.* If you feel sad and alone, listen to the song "No One Is Alone" by Stephen Sondheim from the iconic musical *Into the Woods.* That song is always a healing balm for me.

#5: *This relationship might end.* When I first started setting boundaries, I was so scared because I thought, *I am going to cause this relationship to end.* As if my lack of boundaries is what's holding this thing together?! If someone is your true ally, then they'll want to support you in being your best self. Most people will rise to the occasion of supporting you to get what you need!

Most of my relationships have improved because of healthy boundaries. That said, not all relationships are meant to live on forever, so if setting a boundary leads to a relationship transitioning into its next phase, that may be what's necessary and best for your soul's growth and evolution. Honor every relationship for what it came to teach you, and whether people stay in your life or go on, remember they, too, are learning about who they truly are—in their own, unique way.

My friend Mark Groves authored another favorite quote of mine, "You want to come into my life, the door is open. You want to leave my life, the door is open. Just one request—don't stand at the door, you're blocking traffic."

Codependency

The essence of codependency is, *I can't be okay unless you're okay.* When I am in a codependent relationship with someone, I unconsciously give my power away to that person. I am looking for them to fill a hole that can only be filled when I remember my True Self and my connection to Source. Through codependency, I try to make another human being my Source instead of accessing the power within *me.*

Codependency creates a cloud of confusion as to *where I end and the other person begins.* A codependent dynamic thrives off of zero boundaries, and without conscious awareness, I might quickly lose myself in another person—becoming fixated on them as a means to source my sense of safety and self. Codependency turns us into a puppet controlled by the thoughts, emotions, and behaviors of our partner. If they are high, we are high. If they are low, we are low. If they are loving us, we are loving us. If they are angry with us, we are angry with us. Let me say this right now: you are not responsible for how other people feel about you.

I never identified as codependent. Just didn't click for me. When someone mentioned it, I'd start thinking about something else—as if the person were speaking a language I didn't understand. Then one day, an ex-boyfriend yelled in my face, "You're so fucking codependent, Shannon!" Sometimes relationships can be the loveliest little mirrors, can't they? I loathed such an accusation—and of course, I instantly rejected his erroneous claim! All the while, I was totally hooked into his emotional state, 24/7, as a means to determine my own sense of self. I was losing connection to my True Self with each passing hour of that relationship.

When we unconsciously give so much of our power away to another person, we lose ourselves to the point of wondering, *Who am I without this person? Do I even exist without them?* That's why it can feel so scary to unravel from a codependent partnership.

Here are the steps for confronting codependency with compassion:

1. Ask yourself: *Where am I giving my power away to another person? Where is my mental and emotional health dependent on someone else's mental and emotional state?*

2. Journal: *What would it feel like to be fully responsible for my mental and emotional state? How can I take care of myself first and foremost?*

3. Reflect: *What's one thing I can do right now to set a boundary— no matter how small—to create some space for my own autonomy and agency?*

4. Love: *Think of the child in you who just wants to be loved—who learned to give and receive love in certain ways. Imagine wrapping this child—who will always live within you—with tender loving compassion and care. Try literally hugging and holding yourself.*

Remember that there are even more ways to give and receive love than the ones you learned when you were young. Way more! While shifting a codependent dynamic can feel scary or overwhelming, it is essential for you to stand fully in your power.

Sex for the Soul

It's time for the sex talk! ;) Sex is so outwardly and subtly shamed in our culture that our sexuality is like an uncharted territory—in which our communication skills are dull like butter knives and leave much to be desired when it comes to emotional intimacy and authentic connection in the bedroom. Sex is as human in nature as eating food when hungry, drinking water when thirsty, and dancing when happy. Sex is a holy act of connection! Although, as is evidenced by how much harm is done through unconscious sexual engagement, this is an area that requires much healing and skill building. For many, sex has been a war zone of betrayal, miscommunication, pain, and even violence.

Because the bedroom (or the kitchen counter!) is left out of so many conversations—especially spiritual ones, I want to share a tool that totally changed the way I communicate in sexual relationships. Using this tool in sexual partnerships has improved my communication in all other relationships in my life, as well.

After serving seven years as a team commander in the Israeli Air Force commando unit, Shachar Caspi is now a teacher of sacred sexuality. He works with people to heal their relationship with sexuality and activate exploration and communication through pleasure. Shachar created a communication checklist to use before having any kind of sexual encounter with another person. My personal experience of implementing this—as well as the experiences of my friends, clients, and loved ones—has been nothing short of transformative and inspiring. The response I've received from sharing this tool reminds me how sorely this conversation is needed—to ensure we are honoring ourselves and one another. Not just in sexual encounters, but in all types of relationships. The acronym is B.D.S.M.R.: Boundaries. Desires. Sexually transmitted infections (STIs). Meaning. Relationships.

Next time you're about to get down with someone, I dare you to have this conversation!

Boundaries. What are my boundaries? What are yours?

Example: "I would like to keep our clothes on." Or, "I don't want to have sexual intercourse, but I'm open to X or Y, or I prefer not to X until we establish more trust."

Desires. What are my desires? What are yours?

Example: "I would like you to rub my shoulders. And I want to kiss you."

STIs. When was I last tested, and what were the results? When were you last tested and what were the results?

Example: "I was tested in December, and the results were negative" Or, "I occasionally do get cold sores, but I don't have any right now." Or "I tested positive for chlamydia and I've completed my medication, but I'm due to be retested."

Meaning. What does this sexual encounter mean to me? And to you?

Example: "I know that I care about you, and to me, this means that I am attracted to and respect you. I want to explore more of our relationship potential." Or, "For me, this feels like an exploration of physical pleasure and enjoying this connection fully. I'm not looking for a committed partnership right now."

Relationships. What other significant romantic or sexual relationships do I have in my life? How about you?

Example: "I am single." Or, "I live with my partner of five years, and we have an open agreement. These are the limits I need to share with you." Or, "My husband is pulling up right now. Can he join?"

That last one was a joke. But you never know! And this is why we practice being explicitly honest with one another.

Some of the benefits I've noticed from having the B.D.S.M.R. conversation before sex are increased intimacy, more intentionality, deeper trust, and a sense of empowerment that comes from daring to be myself with a partner. Sex is pure communication, and when you invite the body, mind, and heart into the conversation, you can cocreate something magical with your partner. Give it a try!

Having this conversation, while it can be nerve-racking and vulnerable to initiate, means you get to be yourself. Honesty and being true to yourself is sexy. And if someone is incapable of having this conversation with you, do you really want to be having sex with them? If yes, that's cool—no judgment here! By honoring yourself and your partner in this way, you are building a more trusting relationship with yourself. Now go get after it!!!

CREATE YOUR NEW TEMPLATE

Your relationship with others is based on your relationship with yourself. If you struggle to love yourself, love from others will bounce right off of you. If you struggle to believe in yourself, you won't fully trust people when they believe in you. What you see in others is a reflection of your own inner world—the environment of space within *you*. It's obviously not your fault for having the templates you were given, but it is your responsibility to heal and create something new. You can get—and deserve to have—tons of support, love, cheerleading, and guidance from others as you do this work, *but only you can create something new for yourself.*

Relationships are designed to help you heal. They call up all of the areas within yourself that require more healing so you can become the fullest, most whole expression of who you are. So your soul can awaken. And it is your work—in this body, in this life—to dismantle all of the templates within you that have clouded and confused you from knowing who you are so you can awaken to becoming all that you are, who you have always been, and who you are meant to be.

Relationships show us all the unloved parts of our insides, and they cause us to reckon with the moments when we didn't receive love when we needed it, when we didn't give love when we really wanted to, and all the spaces inside of us now that desire to love and be loved. And through the healing work that occurs through the divine assignments of our relationships, we are called forth to fully realize our unique, creative purpose and expression.

Now it's time to create something new. To harness the power of the lessons you've learned—from joys and disappointments, from lovers and heartbreaks. Rewriting your template will have a ripple effect into all areas of your life. Look back at what you wrote in your journal as the essence of your old template. Take a moment to read it and breathe into it. Feel the body, and any sensation or emotion that comes up as you face it—as you look it dead in the eye.

In your journal, write these five statements, and let the answers flow out of you—through the pen and onto the page. Write as much as you like. Let these words be a healing balm that creates a new narrative for your life. What do you know, deep down, to be true?

I am...

I deserve...

I desire...

I give myself permission to...

The world will benefit from me owning this because...

This is your new template. Reread it to yourself. Notice how it feels. Does it feel real? Does it feel like a pipe dream? What does the old template have to say about the new template?

Now that you've identified what this new template is for yourself, we want to move into the work of owning it, claiming it, and believing it. In the chapters to come, we're going to build upon this new template—so it can gain strength, momentum, and power. So you can trust that this new template is your truth.

You are here to create something in this world that is so uniquely *you*. This is your purpose, and this next phase of our work is about you harnessing your power to build a life of truth. Imagine you can stand on the shoulders of all the lessons your relationships have taught you. What does it feel like to embody this new template? What do you get to create now?

CHAPTER 3

Power Up Your Soul's Purpose

Solar Plexus Chakra, *Manipura*

Color: Yellow

Element: Fire

Body: Gut, stomach, abdominals, lumbar spine, digestion

Emotional Impact: Sense of self, house of the soul, awareness of "I" and "me"

Shadow: Shame

Light: Personal power

Soul Truth: *I know who I am, and I'm ready to activate my soul's purpose.*

Mantra: *Ram* (Bringing the awareness to the navel, repeat "ram"—sounds like mom—out loud or silently eight times before beginning to read this chapter. Sense the energy of power and fire.)

You are a powerhouse. You get to define who you are, who you want to be, what you are capable of, and what you are here to accomplish. But self-doubt and shame can block you from experiencing yourself as the powerhouse that you are. So, let's dive into the core work of developing confidence from the inside out. This chapter is about you—owning your power, tapping into your strength, knowing who you are and what *you* are here to do on this planet. When you're confident in yourself, you can fully embody your power and be a conscious participant in helping others and healing our planet. This world needs *all* of your True, Badass Self to show up now. Buckle up, sweetheart. 'Cause we're about to get *fierce.*

The third chakra, *manipura,* is the solar plexus, and it's through this energy center that we access "the fire in the belly" and harness the heat of fire so we can blaze a trail that is in alignment with our soul's purpose. Developmentally, we are moving from the "we" of the first chakra and the "you and me" of the second chakra to the "me" of the third chakra. The third chakra embodies the energy of a self-confidence that says, "This is me. This is who I am." You know how the planets orbit around the sun? The third chakra helps you find your inner-sun-center, your personal power. The third chakra is "the house of the soul." When this chakra is underactive, you may find yourself playing small and feeling trapped by feelings of unworthiness. When this energy center is overactive, you may find yourself conceited, narcissistic, and hustling to prove your worth. When this energy center is in balance, there is a strong sense of "I am enough." No hiding. No performing. You are present. Connected to your center. You stand your ground with both confidence and humility.

The research of Marvin Oka (2016) from the Australian Spinal Research Foundation teaches how science indicates we actually have three brains—the mind, the heart, and the gut. Because all three have their own intrinsic nervous systems and can learn new information, science defines each as a unique "brain." Oka writes,

"[The gut is how we] find our core identity. What is me, what is not me? This is the domain of the gut brain. It is also responsible for safety and protection. Our gut is extremely important in upholding our immune system, but it also takes care of self-preservation, fear, anxiety, mobility, and action. Gut-based language says things like, 'It takes guts,' or 'Let's do it.'"

This chapter is dedicated to finding your true center so you can experience the confidence of knowing, *I am here, on my path, doing what I need to do to show up for myself and the world. Confidence comes from my core—from honoring my soul's mission and calling.*

To awaken to your soul's purpose, you must know and trust yourself. Before we explore who you truly are and what you really stand for, let's take a look at what gets in the way of you being your badass self.

THE SHADOW OF SHAME

The shadow of the third chakra is shame. Shame blocks us from remembering our inherent power. It's the belief that we are fundamentally bad or broken. It lives in our cells and subconscious minds as "I am not enough." It causes isolation, disconnection, depression, anxiety, suicide, and addiction. At its core, shame is the misperception that we are alone in our suffering and don't deserve love, belonging, and support. How could we possibly be confident in ourselves if we believe who we are—at our core—is bad?

When we're overcome with shame, the voice in our head usually sounds like:

- I am not worthy.

- I don't deserve this.

- What's wrong with me?

- I'm a terrible person.

- I deserve to be alone.

- I'm unlovable.

The nastiest things you could ever say to yourself about yourself... that's shame. And, the most terrible-awful-horrible-no-good thing about shame is it attempts to stop you from showing up, reclaiming your power, and being the badass you are here to be (and already *are*). You don't need to earn your right to show up, be here, shine bright, and kick ass. You're already ready, and only shame would attempt to tell you you're not.

Through her research on shame and vulnerability and in her book *I Thought It Was Just Me* (2007), Dr. Brené Brown teaches the practice of "shame resilience," which she found by identifying the practices of research participants whose lives appeared to be less dictated by shame—who Brené categorized as living "wholehearted" lives. Here are the practices of shame resilience:

1. Identify shame.

2. Recognize the messages underlying shame.

3. Reach out.

4. Speak shame.

Notice when shame is arising within you, and see if you can stand fully in the truth of your experience. Whenever you stay fully present in the moment, shame begins to dissolve and dissipate. The templates you uncovered in the first two chapters can help you recognize the roots of your old shame narratives and the underlying messages. The work is to recognize the presence of shame and to not let it overtake your sense of self-worth.

Shame thrives in secrecy and carries with it this belief that says, *What's wrong with me? I'm so fucked up that I must be the only person going through this right now.* Because of this intense inclination toward isolation and shutting down, reaching out for connection and *speaking shame* are some of the most powerful tools to dissolve it. Connection heals shame—almost instantaneously—because it says, "You are not alone. Me too." There's a great relief that happens when we share our experiences with one another—especially the ones that we think we should *never name or speak about.* And, often when we speak about shame, we hear the ridiculousness of it and see the holes in its logic.

My rule of thumb is if I'm telling myself, "Shannon, you can't talk about this," I know shame must be festering beneath the surface. Reach out and speak the unspeakable, and you'll find yourself letting go of the heaviness that comes from hiding what's truly going on for you underneath the surface.

I remember when I was seventeen, during the weeks leading up to when I came out to my parents, I felt like I was living a lie. I knew I was hiding my authentic self from them, and it felt terrible. Like I was carrying around a ton of bricks. Even though my mom once told me while we were watching *Oprah,* "If you ever realize you're gay, I'll always love you!" I still had a ton of fear about how they'd react. Like the emo teenager that I was (and still kinda am), I gathered my mom and dad around the table in our dining room and dimmed the lights on the chandelier so the light would reflect my somber moodiness. I was nervous and scared.

When my parents responded with such support saying, "We'll always love you—no matter what. Let's go out to dinner!" I was so relieved. Instantly, the heaviness lifted from my body, and I felt light because I dared to tell them who I am. When we share who we truly are with people, we create the opportunities for real connection…to be truly seen. Shame cannot survive in the presence of connection. I realize I'm incredibly privileged because my parents accepted my sexuality and chose to love an aspect of me that they were unfamiliar with. For the moments when you dared to be yourself and the other person didn't reach back to love you and *see you*, your courage was enough. You are enough. Keep going—keep being you, and you will find love, connection, and belonging.

The greatest gift you can ever give or receive is the gift of being proud of who you are. The shame-induced belief that you are broken and unworthy of love and connection will *never be true*. You are good, whole, perfect as you are, and *totally* worthy of all the love in the world. The voice of shame may never disappear completely, but your belief in shame's false messages will lessen with practice. Each time you practice shame resilience and remember your inherent worthiness, you experience more of your True Self.

PERSONAL POWER

It's possible you might not realize how much power you actually have. I know I didn't. Personal power is your ability to make conscious choices that honor your truth and enhance your life force energy. Harnessing your personal power means your energy is strong, your actions are precise and clear, and you have a sense of who you are. If you feel disempowered, you may be giving power away to someone or something outside of you. When this happens, your energy leaks and your fire dampens. Your job is to learn to stoke the flame and wield your power.

In Hinduism, there are two deities—one masculine and one feminine—whose union is said to be responsible for the whole Universe. Shiva is the force that makes up all of the "stuff," the content of the Universe, and Shakti's dynamic potency makes it possible for all the "stuff" to come forth into manifestation. Shakti is power, ability, strength, effort, energy, and capability. It allows your energy to reach far beyond your physical body.

Have you ever felt someone walk into a room, and you say, "Who's *that?*" Think of someone whose presence you can palpably feel. I once stood front row center at a Beyoncé concert. In a moment I'll never forget, Queen Bey sang directly into my iPhone camera. Then, she directed her focus to the back of the sold-out 19,000-seat stadium. I felt Shakti, indeed! Beyoncé's energy radiated through the entire space.

Harnessing Shakti energy helps you cut the cords of attachment that are causing you to give your power away. So you can fully embody the power that is your birthright. Each of the next practices invites you to be in the moment with attentiveness and presence so you can sense your power and harness your strength.

Stop the Energy Leaks

The fundamental question of the third chakra is, *What are you giving your life energy to?* When you unconsciously give your power away to someone or something outside of you, you actually lose prana—your life force energy. Imagine you're trying to heat up your house in the winter, but you leave a big door open; the cold will get inside, and it will take way more energy to heat the house. *Notice for the next few days: Which choices deplete you, and which choices give you life?* When you make choices that are life-giving, you start to become an actual powerhouse—an energetic forcefield of potent and palpable life energy. If there's an area of your life where there's an energy leak, then it's time to cut the cords so you can reclaim what's yours.

We so often give our power away because we *think* we have no other choice. One of the most common ways we give our power away is through our attention. We focus on gossip, news, drama, social media, or other people's problems as a means to tune out or numb ourselves from feeling whatever it is that we're feeling. Through distraction, we become depleted. It takes intention and heat to own your power because you are choosing to take full responsibility for your energetic force field. With great power comes great "response-ability."

Response-Ability

"Response-ability" is your ability to respond. When you practice response-ability, you are conscious of your power, and when you default to reactivity, you are asleep to your power. All of us go through this process of floating between sleep and awake. Practice patience and compassion with yourself as you become more aware. The gift of becoming more response-able is that you get to have more of a say in the matters of your life. In any moment, you can remember your power to choose.

Here are ways we stay asleep to our power:

- Waiting and expecting someone else to do the work

- Cynicism: "It is the way it is"

- Tolerating bad behavior from others

- Staying in a toxic job or relationship because "we have to"

- Alcohol and drugs

- Outsourcing our power to others

- Distractions that keep us playing small

- Making choices that dishonor our soul's needs.

Awaken to your response-ability! Your actions—no matter how big or small—have a magnificent ripple effect into all areas of your life. In every situation of your life, you can ask yourself, *By making this choice, am I reclaiming my personal power, or am I giving my personal power away?*

UNDERSTANDING PERSONAL POWER VS. SYSTEMIC POWER

If you've ever felt like you don't actually have a choice, that you just "had to do" something and you didn't have a say in the matter, you may have either given your personal power away *or* had your personal power taken away from you. In both cases, you're off your center.

A long history of oppression and abuse of systemic power has caused people in our society to have less freedom and agency. Because of systemic injustice, we operate in a society that privileges and uplifts some folks while oppressing and marginalizing others. No one should suggest that the playing field is level and that systemic power doesn't play a role in our relationship to personal power. Because it does. Marginalized people all over our world—women, Black, Indigenous, and People of Color (BIPOC), folks with differing levels of physical ability, undocumented immigrants, and LGBTQ folks, to name a few—have had power stripped from them for centuries while others capitalize off of their oppression through maintaining the "status quo." If you have been harmed by systemic injustice, it's essential to acknowledge how systemic power plays a role in the internalization of self-doubt and your relationship to your inherent personal power. In too many spirituality and personal development spaces, I've seen responsibility put onto marginalized folks when these types of questions get directed to them: "Well, what is your role in manifesting this in your life? You are the creator of your life!" Or, "What part of you keeps attracting these oppressive circumstances?" While there may be a time and place for these types of conversations, it is not appropriate to ask someone with a systemic (or literal) knee on their neck, "What did you do to create this?" This is a harmful and retraumatizing form of spiritual gaslighting, and we need to call it out when we see it so we can deal with the ways in which systemic power continues to perpetuate the upliftment of some at the expense of others. We are ALL responsible for dismantling oppressive systems both within ourselves and in our communities. This is essential to our personal and collective healing and liberation.

And, while systemic power may influence your relationship to your personal power, the truth is we *all* have access to our inner strength. And despite what has occurred leading up to this moment now, you are the only one who can take your personal power back. You can't always stop your power from being taken away, but learning to reclaim and embody your personal power is your birthright. Even amidst moments of tortuous adversity and injustice, the human spirit has the capacity to find light within the shadows of these experiences *and* to discover ways to bring those shadow experiences to the light— for the greater good of our collective awakening. Regardless of the hand you've been dealt, you deserve to rise up and know the full capacity of your badass strength.

GO WITH YOUR GUT

I was in a relationship once where I had this sense—this gut knowing—that my partner was cheating on me. For almost a year, my body was telling me something was up. I didn't have tangible proof, but the feeling was so strong, it burned in my gut. On several occasions, I approached him and said, "Hey...I'm not sure why I feel this way...but I have this strong sense that _____ is happening. Is this true?"

Time after time, he would lie, get angry, blame me, and point the finger, "You're crazy! What's wrong with you? Why can't you trust me?" Despite giant, billowy red flags, I believed him. *I wanted to believe him.* Every time we would fight, I would blame myself.... I started to believe I was crazy.

Until one night, after we had moved to Los Angeles, coleased a car and an apartment, purchased furniture, and even gotten a cell phone plan together, I had that burning feeling in my gut again. As I sat with it, I hesitated to bring it up to him because I knew it might cause another fight—he'd get mad, and I'd end up feeling guilty. I brought it up anyway; my body almost forced me to press the issue. And on that night, unlike so many other nights preceding it, he admitted to cheating on me.

This relationship carried with it so many lessons for me, but the biggest one was the discovery of the *very real* power of my gut intuition. It turned out that *every single time* I had a feeling that something was off, my gut was right. And every time I believed his narrative and devalued my own gut truth, I gave more of my personal power away. I was losing so much power in that relationship, I was losing myself, and the more I lost myself, the more I became a puppet—tied up in a narrative that was untrue.

For so many of us, we learn how to reclaim our personal power through, first, giving too much of it away. We need to lose it to learn the lesson of reclaiming it. The moment my ex started to come clean about all of the things he had been lying to me about, I literally felt my body start to recharge with the power it had lost. As the clouds of delusion started to part, I realized the degree to which I had been living my life based on his lie. *It cost me actual life energy to suppress and avoid my gut's true knowing.* For me, it was through this experience that the expression "go with your gut" graduated from being some positive affirmation that people say to becoming a real-life practice that now informs how I move through the world, trusting my truth.

I invite you to share in this lesson with me—to really commit to develop and strengthen your relationship with your gut. Listen to its wisdom! Sometimes, it goes against what is "logical" and "makes sense" because it holds a deeper, embodied truth and wisdom from all five koshas.

What is your gut telling you? It's always communicating. Learn to listen to the sensation, the information, the signposts...and most importantly, learn to trust its guidance. There is useful information being provided to you in every single moment, and your job is to learn to listen to this "brain" that operates differently than the mind. Try not to "figure it out" on a mental level, but rather, get curious by asking questions like,

What is my gut telling me?

What does my body know to be true?

What happens when I follow the wisdom of my gut—even when it feels scary and doesn't make 100 percent logical sense?

A potent way to get to know your gut is when you become triggered by something.

WORK WITH THE TRICKY TRIGGERS

A trigger occurs when you are physically, mentally, or emotionally disrupted by an external stimulus—be it a person, circumstance, or event—and your sympathetic nervous system is stimulated into the fight, flight, or freeze response to the point of dysregulation. When you are triggered, your attention becomes almost fully—if not completely—enveloped by that which triggered you.

As I learned from Somatic Experiencing therapist and trauma-informed yoga teacher, Hala Khouri, author of *Peace from Anxiety,* when we are triggered, our power gets pinged away from our center and becomes displaced onto whatever, or whoever, triggered us. In other words, if you are triggered by someone else's actions, the location of your core center moves from your body over to the person whose actions triggered you. Your center is now outside of yourself. So, the tendency when you are triggered is to become fixated on the other person because you feel energetically hooked and tied to them.

You are dysregulated, and without consciousness and tools, you unconsciously become a puppet, their marionette. The other person's thoughts, words, and actions are like strings pulling at you. You may obsessively try to change them or get them to behave differently. But the more you try to control someone else, the more you lose personal power.

You can't change someone else, so the best thing you can do for yourself (and the other person) in these moments is take a step back and find your center. There were so many moments when I wanted my ex-boyfriend to behave differently, but my obsession with his behavior was knocking me off my center. Here's how you can bring your center back from that other person or external circumstance and bring it home to you.

RECLAIM YOUR POWER BY CENTERING

The fastest way to reclaim your power is to make choices that strengthen you. Centering is the practice of energetically reclaiming your power—right now in this moment. Other actions may be necessary down the line to fully reclaim power in your external life, but centering allows you to stop energy leaks and reclaim your power *right now*. You can do it almost anywhere. Let's give it a try:

Flatten the palm of each hand and bring the fingers together so there's no space between your fingers. Imagine each hand is a blade and the pinky finger is the sharp edge. Now, take your hands and begin to chop the air around the body. Yep. Chop chop! Imagine you are cutting all the cords of the external world—all your responsibilities, relationships, attachments, to-do lists, everything! Chop in front of your body, on the sides of your body, and even behind your head and back. Keep chopping as if you can feel the puppet strings of attachment to anything outside yourself being cut.

Then, stop and close your eyes. As you close your outer eyes to the external world, imagine your inner eye opening. Tune your awareness inward. Notice if you can relax any tension in the body that is unnecessary, perhaps from a previous moment or interaction.

Direct your attention to your navel and feel it moving out on the inhalation and moving toward the spine on the exhalation. As you breathe, see a warm, healing, yellow, light energy at the center of your core—like the fire of the sun. As your body breathes, imagine the breath fanning the flames of this inner sunlight as the light begins to glow and grow bigger and bigger. With every exhale, imagine one more layer of attachment being shed—releasing any tension as if a ship is being sent off to sea, moving far away from your body. With every inhale, feel the power of the sun growing stronger in your center.

Feel and breathe into your center. Feel how your life energy is self-contained and self-sufficient. Take a few moments to continue to breathe into your center and feel this light grow and flow—from the inside out.

EMBRACE YOUR EGO (AND LET IT GO!)

The ego gets a bad rap, and it's true…it can cause a lot of problems. But the ego is neither good nor bad. It's your identity, your sense of self. The ego gets us into trouble when we let it run the show of our lives; an unchecked ego wants to enhance its identity regardless of the cost, harm, or impact. The nature of an ego in charge is *I want more!* More money, sex, power, food, booze, TV, social media followers. More. More. More. More. More. The ego is obsessed with wanting but is never satiated by having. For this reason, it often feeds shame's pesky "never enough" narrative. Shame can trigger the ego to seek and keep seeking until we drive ourselves into a ditch of despair.

But the ego also plays an important role in our human experience. Without it, we wouldn't have a sense of self—there'd be no "me." If I didn't have an ego, I wouldn't write this book. It's the ego that says, "You have something to say. Write!" or "You've got a job to do. You're the one to do it." When the ego is in check and we have a healthy relationship to it, it supports us to be on purpose. Instead of being driven by it, we utilize it as a tool to be of service to the greater good. An ego in service of Spirit is a powerful force for transformation and healing. An ego in service of itself—with no awareness of its connection to the Whole—can be a dangerous weapon and inflict unconscious harm. When your ego is in service of itself, you may find yourself caring about:

- How you look to others from the outside

- How much money you make

- Checking off the boxes of societal norms

- Acquiring more

- How things look "on paper."

When the ego is not in check, we tend to either shrink and play small *or* we puff up and overcompensate. When I studied theater in college, my acting teacher and voice coach Elizabeth "Lizzie" Ingram taught us about two qualities to become aware of as we set out to truthfully play a character: "Denial" and "Bluff." You can become aware of these qualities based on how a person physically holds and expresses themselves.

In denial, the chest caves in, the shoulders sag forward, and the head shrinks to the floor—as if to say, "Don't look at me. I have nothing to offer. I am small."

In bluff, the shoulders go back, the chest puffs up, the nose points toward the sky—as if to say, "Don't you know who I am? I'm more important than you. I am a very big deal."

The work of an actor is to embody their character truthfully. Your work is to embody yourself truthfully. Denial and bluff are masks that hide your truth, and if you hide who you are, you are essentially robbing yourself and the world of your most valuable resource: *you!*

In her book *Daring Greatly* (2012), Brené Brown shares one of her personal mantras, "Don't shrink. Don't puff up. Just stand your sacred ground." This mantra is the essence of what Lizzie taught us, and it's a powerful tool to check in with when you may find yourself in puffing up (bluff) or shrinking (denial). Can you, as Brené says, stand your sacred ground? Unmasked. Present. Aware. Available. Neutral. Ready. Here. Begin to notice yourself in your life as you move into denial and bluff. We all do it. What happens when you stand your sacred ground and stay true to your center?

I remember the day I went to the "Deepak Homebase" in New York City to interview Deepak Chopra on my podcast "SoulFeed." I was sitting outside his office with my cohost Alex, waiting for him to finish his previous meeting. In just a few minutes, I'd be sitting at Deepak's desk interviewing one of the greatest spiritual leaders of our time! I was giddy with excitement...but also very nervous. My ego was going crazy. I was twenty-eight, "SoulFeed" was only a few months old, and I remember vacillating between two thoughts: (1) *Who do I think I am to interview Deepak Chopra?* and (2) *OMG! I am so fucking badass! I am interviewing Deepak Chopra!* What was really at the root of these two thoughts was (1) *I'm not good enough to interview Deepak,* and (2) *I am a bigger, better person because I am interviewing Deepak.*

In the first thought, I shrunk, and in the second, I puffed up. The vulnerable truth is in the middle...in the label-less space. When the ego tricks us into thinking we're smaller or bigger than other people, we get stuck in an identity—a falsehood, a misperception. When we stand our sacred ground, we show up in presence. We can bring our unfiltered soul self—our truth—to the table of collaboration. Standing your sacred ground and being unmasked by the ego's labels can be scary, clunky, awkward, uncomfortable, and even terrifying. But the sacred middle ground is the birthplace of confidence— because you're daring to be the real you.

Your ego will always be with you—and it has both shadow and light. The more you are conscious of how it operates, the less you will be controlled by it and the more it can support your true calling. The question is, Can you use your ego to be of service to your soul's purpose? When you do this, you begin to ride a wave of purpose that is much bigger than you. You can use your human life to connect to something greater and more fulfilling, purposeful, aligned, abundant, and true than you could ever imagine!

YOUR DHARMA CODE

Your dharma is your unique calling, your reason for being here on this planet at this time—it's your soul's purpose. Each of us has a dharma, and it lives in us like a code. It's informed by your life experience, but it's also deeply embedded in your soul. The soul has a thirst to get on an aligned path of personal expression in this life—to be useful, purposeful, and of service.

When you ask the question, *How is my individual soul called to be of service to the greater good?* you are tapping into your dharma, and you can harness your personal Shakti power to be of service to your dharma. So, how do you discover your dharma? Here are five tools for you to unlock your unique dharma code.

Use Shame as the Doorway to Purpose

Your deepest shadow can actually awaken you to the power of your light. Through having the courage to reckon with shame, you move closer to your purpose. Your purpose is not something outside of you—*you are your purpose.* When shame sends you into a spiral, your dharma calls you forth—out of your small self so you can be your True Self. By embracing shame instead of turning your back on it, you can harness the fire within to blaze a new trail in your life. Ask yourself and journal:

What is an area where I feel—or have felt—shame?

How might healing my relationship to this shame enable me to be of service in a bigger way?

Who do I get to become when I believe I am not only worthy but needed on this planet? What do I get to create?

What would I do right now if I trusted in my worthiness and value?

Your purpose is
not something
outside of you. You
are your purpose.

♡

Look at What You Love

What makes you come alive? Just as it is the flower's destiny to bloom and offer its nectar to the bees and all who come to enjoy its fragrance, it is your job to listen to what brings you joy. Sometimes, when we think of purpose, we think solely of career, and while some people earn money doing their dharma, you never "clock out" of your soul's purpose. *Your dharma is who you are.* It's bigger than one role you play or job you have. It's how you are called to show up for your lover... and your boss. For your best friend...and the homeless person asking you for money on the street. For the grocery store clerk...and the person writing you a check. It transcends any one aspect of who you are, and it floods every area of your life with a desire to be of service.

What is something in your life that you really love to do? It might be something basic or mundane that is actually so satisfying, like working on a puzzle or making soup for a sick loved one. Or, it might be a significant leap or goal, like raising $10,000 for a cause you care about or running for political office. Ask yourself and journal:

What are one to three activities I absolutely love to do? That bring me joy—just for the sake of being joyful?

What feels joyful about each of these activities?

What qualities are awakened within me when I do them?

Acknowledge What You're Good At

What are you good at? For me, I've always loved writing. In seventh grade, I was weirdly obsessed with diagramming sentences— where you identify the subject of a sentence, the verb, adjectives, adverbs, and so forth. Wielding words as an art of communication has always been fun for me and something I've felt a sense of excellence and flow around. So I knew I always wanted to write a book. And, here we are.

What is something you're really good at? Maybe it's making sandwiches! Don't *prejudge* whether what you're good at is "useful" or "useless." Doing so castrates the possibility of exploration. Just acknowledge, *Hey! Yeah, I'm really good at* _____. Ask yourself and journal:

What is one skill I am really good at?

What do I feel in my body when I do this skill?

How does it feel to offer this gift to, or share this experience with, others?

What feedback—if any—have I received from others about this skill?

Recall a Time When You Felt On Purpose

When was a time when you felt truly "on purpose"? Maybe it was a time when you were super young. There may be several things that come to mind or just a few. In any area of your life, reflect back to a time when you felt "in the flow"—that you were exactly where you were meant to be. Perhaps you felt helpful and useful. That you were uniquely positioned to be of service in some way.

I remember the feeling of riding in AIDS/LifeCycle, a seven-day bike ride from San Francisco to Los Angeles to raise money and awareness to end the AIDS epidemic. I rode with my team of college friends and alongside HIV "positive pedalers"; we biked 545 miles with a shared and common goal. The feeling of purpose and community was electrifying. If I dropped my helmet, at least five people would go to pick it up. If someone's tire went flat, it would be fixed within ten minutes. I felt so much pride to be a part of this cause —raising millions of dollars to support people with—and prevent— HIV/AIDS. I remember feeling like there was *no place else I'd rather be than doing exactly that.*

This doesn't have to be a "big deal" thing, but what's most important is that you felt connected to a purpose greater than you and you were aware of your unique contribution to that larger purpose. Ask yourself and journal:

> *Looking back on my life thus far, what gives me the greatest feeling of accomplishment and significance?*

Discover Your Why Statement

In his TED talk and book *Start with Why* (2009), Simon Sinek encourages us to dive deeper into our purpose by looking at not just *what* we do and not just *how* we do it but *why* we do what we do. Just like Anamaya kosha, the Physical body, the "what" of our lives is the most external. You may call yourself a lawyer or a teacher. This is your "what." The "how" goes a little deeper into your unique style or approach. You may use humor to educate in your classroom. Or you may write poetry to express your feelings about politics. Your "why" is the deepest core level of what drives you. It's your dharma! And like your dharma, your why is not something you make up or create; it lives within you like a code that you are destined to crack, unlock, and ignite forth into the world. Ultimately, all of our collective "whys" are designed to awaken us to being of service to support our planet in healing and becoming whole.

In my Illuminate Your Purpose—Career Manifestation course, I teach students to discover their *why* statement—which acts as a written, verbal reminder of *what really drives them*. Here's how to discover your why.

Look at your answers. Review your responses to this section's journal prompts that identify your healing through shame, what you really love, your gifts and skills, and a time when you felt right "on purpose."

Identify the common theme. For example, for me:

- I've worked quite a bit on healing the shame that says, "Shannon, when you speak your truth, you might hurt people."

- I really love travel adventures with friends.

- I'm really good at using words to articulate ideas.

- I felt so incredibly on purpose when I rode my bike from San Francisco to Los Angeles with AIDS/LifeCycle.

So my theme is *using my voice to energize and motivate people to come together around a common cause.* Find a common theme in your answers, some kind of overlap. This does *not* have to be perfectly clear. This stage of the process can be messy.

Ask WHY? Look at *your* theme. Ask yourself these questions, and journal your answers to each. *Please note: Don't overthink this! Notice your breath, get your pen on the page, and let the wisdom pour out of you. See what is revealed.*

- Looking at your theme, answer this question, *Why is this even important to me?*

- Looking at your new answer, now ask, *Why does this matter?*

- Looking at your new answer, now ask, *Why do I really care about this?*

- Looking at your new answer, now ask, *Why is this so important for the betterment of the world?*

Create your *why* statement. Your *why* statement is the root of why you do what you do. It's what you really care about—on the deepest level. Look at all of your answers to the above "why" questions. Circle any common words or themes that you see from repeatedly asking why. As an example, my why statement is, "*I am a light that is here to illuminate the power that already exists within every human being I come into contact with.*" Your *why* is simple, and through this exercise, you're doing your best to use words to name something that is truly unnameable. It goes deeper than language. Try not to get too caught up in the mind around this and instead, trust in the themes revealing themselves. Trust that the answers are already alive and present within you and your only work is to allow your why to be given a voice and space to fully express itself.

Live your *why*. When you know your dharma—your *why*—you can fact-check all of your actions and choices to assess whether or not you are in alignment with the calling of your soul. Taking aligned action is a key practice for you to bring the energy of your dharma into the world—and to manifest your purpose in your life in a practical way. And every time you take an aligned action that honors your why, you build confidence in your True Self! Your *why* may be something that you refine and clarify as you move throughout your life, but its essence does not change. It stretches across the span the whole of your life.

The first three chakras are the lower chakras, which are "of the earth." These energy centers influence how you move through your life—based on your upbringing, your relationships, and your connection to your ego self. In the coming chapters, we move into the upper chakras, which connect our earthly purpose to a higher spiritual purpose. As we move into the fourth chakra, we're going to explore the power of emotions and the role the heart plays in waking us up to the truth.

CHAPTER 4

Let Your Heart Lead

Heart Chakra, *Anahata*

Color: Green

Element: Air

Body: Heart, circulatory system, lungs, respiratory system, rib cage

Emotional Impact: Emotional intelligence, the ability to move energy throughout the body, compassion, Wisdom body

Shadow: Grief and resentment

Light: Divine love

Soul Truth: *I feel it to heal it.*

Mantra: *Yam* (Bringing the awareness to the heart center, repeat yam—sounds like "yum"—out loud or silently eight times before beginning to read this chapter. Sense the energy of tender love.)

The heart—your emotional power center—is where you feel the full spectrum of human emotion and cultivate compassion and empathy for yourself and other beings. Emotions awaken your soul to its purpose and truth. They help you feel all the areas within yourself that require emotional healing and empowerment in order for your dharma to come to life. Your heart amplifies your purpose and connects you to an unseen, but deeply felt, level of power and wisdom within you.

While the third chakra—your gut—is the center of your physical "human" self, the fourth chakra—your heart—is the center of your spiritual "being" self. The third chakra connects you to your worldly purpose, and the fourth chakra connects you to your spiritual purpose. Your heart is drawn to its higher calling because it's the closest to the center of the soul; it's the doorway to the Wisdom and Bliss bodies.

The element of the fourth chakra is air—like the air being breathed by your lungs. The lungs surround the heart, and as they fill up with oxygen, the lungs gently press against and massage the heart. The heart and the lungs are lifelong cuddle buddies—wrapping each other in oxygen and love. The fire of the solar plexus chakra cannot exist without the air of the heart chakra because it's oxygen in the air that allows fire to exist! We can't see oxygen, but the presence of fire proves it's there. In the same way, the fiery motivation to be in alignment with your soul purpose would not exist without the emotions and desires of the heart.

All emotions, the bitter and the sweet—love, compassion, empathy, ecstasy, joy, grief, sadness, heartache, guilt, shame, and fear—are felt in the heart. It's through the heart that you receive and let go, both emotionally and physically.

Linda Graham, marriage and family therapist and author of *Bouncing Back: Rewiring Your Brain For Maximum Resilience and Well-Being* (2013), writes, "The warm, safe touch of our hand on our heart center begins to activate the release of oxytocin, the brain's hormone of safety and trust, bonding and belonging, calm and connect. Warm, safe touch anywhere that feels comfortable on our body can release the oxytocin, but there are neural cells around the heart that communicate directly with the brain and more quickly begin the activation of the release." The arms are extensions of the heart. They allow you to give and receive throughout your life, and you can use them to recharge and give back to yourself. Try this exercise to tap into your heart energy and get some oxytocin flowing.

> Take just a brief moment of pause to place your nondominant hand directly on your heart and your dominant hand on top of that one. Feel your hands circling and cycling this heart energy back into yourself in a gesture of recharging, restoring, replenishing, and renewing. Notice your breathing and feel the connection between the hands and the chest. As the body inhales, feel the chest rising into the hands. As the body exhales, feel the hands softening into the chest. For a few breaths, notice this connection to your own heart. If it's comfortable for you, close your eyes and listen to your breath and your heart.

It's through feeling
and riding the waves
of our emotions that
we discover the truth
of who we are.

♡

THE DYNAMIC DUO: MIND AND HEART

For so many of us, the heart is uncharted territory...the "Wild Wild West." We're taught to undervalue the heart's wisdom and to overvalue the mind's strategy and logic. So many of us are hungry for tools to powerfully deal with our emotions so we can harness the power of the heart to its fullest potential. It can feel vulnerable to share our true emotions—especially when we don't fully understand them. And yet, the heart is the space where our deepest truth resides. It's how we meaningfully connect to others, heart to heart.

> Piglet: *How do you spell love?*
>
> Pooh: *You don't spell it, you feel it.*
>
> —A. A. Milne, *Winnie-the-Pooh* (1926)

To protect ourselves from the vulnerability of feeling our feelings, the mind attempts to master and control the heart. But the thing is... as Pooh points out, the heart is not ruled by mental logic. Because the mind speaks the language of thought and the heart speaks the language of emotion, the mind often struggles to "make sense" of the heart. Here's the thing: To build a trusting relationship with your heart, the heart does not need to be understood or "figured out." It needs to be felt, honored, and expressed. The feelings, longings, and desires of the heart will not always be understood—at the level of the thinking mind. *And they don't need to be.*

Remember: The heart is the one pumping the blood to the brain...not the other way around. Our society emphasizes its value on mental intelligence, strategy, cost-benefit analysis, quarterly earnings, productivity over humanity. And so we are conditioned to overunderstand, strategize, and manipulate our way through our lives. Overunderstanding can be just another way of avoiding the emotions that reside in the heart. I catch myself doing this. I try to "think" my way out of feeling. But the great paradox is that it's through feeling and riding the waves of our emotions that we discover the truth of who we are.

Letting the mind run the show without integrating the heart's wisdom and longings may lead to some level of worldly success, but it rarely—if ever—leads to deep soul fulfillment. Because the heart transcends the logic of the mind, the intelligence of the heart is often written off as "emotional," "woo-woo," "not useful," "irrational," or "crazy." This is yet another way that toxic patriarchal culture attempts to disconnect us from our inner power. In reality, just as the gut is considered a brain, so is the heart. By overvaluing the mind and undervaluing the heart, we bypass the heart's true wisdom.

Of course, the mind undoubtedly helps us to survive and create amazing things in this world! But it's better positioned on the *passenger side of your best friend's ride* rather than in the driver's seat. Imagine this: Your body is the car, your heart is your best friend driving, and your mind is in the passenger seat. While the mind may be scared to let the heart drive the car of your life, the heart is determined to carry you toward your soul's next lesson. Where the mind says, "No, I don't wanna go!!!" the heart says, "Take me, I'm ready!"

The costs of being disconnected from—and numb to—the truth that lives within the cavernous walls of your heart are very high. By cutting yourself off from your capacity to fully feel, you distance yourself from your truth. To know and honor your truth on a deep soul level, you want to learn to let your heart lead and let the mind be a useful partner and support system. Trusting your heart can feel scary because it won't always make sense. The heart asks that we open ourselves up to the full human experience—and to allow the soul to fully awaken.

Steve Jobs said in his famous commencement speech at Stanford University (2005), "You can't connect the dots looking forward; you can only connect them looking backwards. So you have to trust that the dots will somehow connect in your future. You have to trust in something—your gut, destiny, life, karma, whatever." One of my favorites. I'd like to add a little flavor to this. *The mind* can only connect the dots looking back. But the heart actually can receive intelligence *in advance*. As you discover, for yourself, the benefits of listening to your heart, it becomes more natural to let it lead.

Here's a Tibetan heart *kriya* to help us to soften and feel the vibration—the aliveness—of the heart. Kriya is Sanskrit for action, effort, or deed—a practice intended to lead you toward a specific result.

You can sit in the position you are now reading in, or you can lie down. Take a deep breath into your heart. Exhale an audible, sweet sigh of relief—feeling the vibration of your exhale right in the heart center. Do this eight more times, and with each exhale, make the sigh a little bit sweeter...as if you were moving deeper into the space of your heart. As you exhale, notice if you can feel the mind letting go and passing the torch of power to the heart. Sense that each exhaling sigh allows you to feel the tenderness of your own heart. Once you've completed about ten heart sighs of relief, sit in stillness for a moment and listen to your heart. Notice if you can feel, hear, or sense the pulsation of your heartbeat coursing through your entire body. Notice what it feels like to bring your full attention to your heart space.

This stillness is the truth of who you are.

YOU ARE NOT YOUR EMOTIONS

On a windy or stormy day, you don't confuse yourself with the storm. You know that you are *in* a storm—experiencing it as it passes. When you experience intense emotions, you're experiencing an emotional storm. But the emotional storm isn't who you are. You want to let yourself *experience* your emotions while remembering your emotions are not who you are.

Emotions are energy in motion. E-motion. They're meant to move through you, be fully felt, and be let go. If you're in a situation where it's "not okay" to fully feel or express your emotion and there's no outlet for the emotion to release, this energy gets trapped in the body. This suppression builds up as stuck energy in the body, which leads to tension and eventually disease. It becomes trapped in the psyche in the form of unfinished soul business.

Just as gusts of wind have the power to move rocks and purify the quality of air, emotions are powerful tools for cleansing and transformation. I know that when I don't want to feel an emotion, I'm usually resisting the transformation that the emotion carries along with it. Your emotions may help you see something in a new way, give you access to more empathy and compassion, change your perspective completely, remind you of the impermanence of life, and/or wake you up to a deeper spiritual truth within yourself.

And yet, for so many of us, we're afraid to feel. We fear the power of our emotions, and so we attempt to shut off the valve in order to stop them from wiping us out. Repressing emotions can cause heaviness and depression—a cloud that blocks you from experiencing your true nature. Overidentifying with emotions can cause you to lose yourself in the story about the emotion. Either way, you end up stuck, pulled away from the center of your True Self.

When I want to stay the same and I resist transformation, I'll try to distract myself from feeling the feelings. I don't want to go "there," so I try to control the emotion instead of allowing it. It's as if a plane is trying to take off, but I'm lying on the runway in front of the plane on my back, saying, "Nooooo! I don't wanna go!!!!!" Like all emotions, the plane will eventually take off. So, I best learn how to get on board and ride the wave of emotion to my next destination.

BREATHE AND FEEL

Emotions are incredibly powerful amplifiers of energy. They run from our hearts through our whole bodies like electrical currents causing us to feel. Without emotion, life would be incredibly boring! Every time you breathe an inhale, your lungs and heart receive new life in the form of oxygen. Every time you release an exhale, your lungs and heart release old energy. Each inhale is literally a birth of new possibility... always followed by an exhale of death and letting go. *Inhale. Exhale.*

Breathing is the means through which you can ride the waves of your emotions. *Inhale to feel. Exhale to release.* According to the *Oxford English Dictionary*, "inspire" comes from the Latin *inspirare*, which means "to breathe or blow into." "The word was originally used of a divine or supernatural being, in the sense '[to] impart a truth or idea to someone.'" "Expire" comes from the Latin *expirare*, which means to "breathe out." With each breath, there is both inspiration and expiration. The breath reveals the constant presence of movement—the transition happening in each and every moment.

If you don't feel safe to feel your emotions or you were taught that it's not okay to express yourself authentically when you were younger, you may hold your breath when a big, intense emotion comes up. When you hold your breath, tension stops the flow of emotion, which is often an attempt to stop yourself from feeling. You might feel tightness in your jaw. When you stop yourself from inhaling and feeling the fullness of the emotion, you also stop yourself from exhaling and getting the benefit of release. This is how we get stuck. Sometimes, emotions can be so suppressed that we don't even know they're there.

By cultivating more awareness of your body, you can feel the clues that the body gives you in the form of sensation. Learning to be present while you feel your emotions increases your ability to harness the power of your heart. When an intense emotion arises, here's what to do:

Notice it. *"I notice I am getting frustrated."*

Feel it. *Feel the sensations. What are the physical sensations felt by the body—as a result of this emotion?*

Process it. *Where is this coming from? What story is the mind making up about this emotion? What is this emotion here to help me remember? Processing may include practices such as exercising, journaling, meditating, or punching a pillow as hard as you can.*

Let it go. *Exhale and imagine the emotion moving through you. Journal and brain dump all the thoughts.*

N.F.P.L. Notice. Feel. Process. Let go.

When you're in the process stage, don't get too caught up in the narrative of figuring out why you feel the way you feel. Sometimes, if you get obsessed with figuring out why you feel a certain way, you can actually get stuck in a loop of mental fixation that prevents you from *feeling it* and *letting it go.* You don't need to understand all of your emotions. That would take so much work...trying to analyze every single emotion that comes through you throughout the day. Remember: Emotions don't need to be understood as much as they need to be felt.

In order to heal whatever is bubbling up to the surface, you've gotta feel it. The sooner you feel, the sooner you can heal. And the more effectively the energy can move.

Owning the Shadow Emotions

We're taught what to think, what to say, how to behave, what to wear, what to eat, who to marry.... But we're not taught how to feel.

For so many of us, we weren't given spaces where it was acceptable and encouraged to feel the full color spectrum of our emotions. And because of this, we didn't learn to speak the language of the heart. If listening to your heart feels new, it can be scary to move deeper into inquiry.

You must create, for yourself, the space to feel. Only you can notice, feel, process, and let go of your feelings. No one else can do it for you. To be emotionally empowered in your heart, you must take full responsibility for the experience you are having. I know this can be difficult sometimes. Taking responsibility may sound like *I am the one experiencing this emotion, but this emotion is not who I am. I feel energy moving through me. I am the responsible steward of how this energy gets moved and released.*

When an emotion is unbearable or nearly impossible to deal with, you might lash out or blame someone else, saying, "*You* are the reason I am feeling this way! This is your fault!!!" When you are at a heightened emotional peak, it can be tempting to discharge the energy onto someone else. It's important to know that, while someone else's words or actions may have triggered an emotional response in you, you are responsible for the energy that's moving through you. Your greatest power lies in your ability to be a responsible steward of the energy you embody.

Learning to paint with your emotional color palette in a way that heals instead of harms yourself and those around you is a profound artform worthy of consistent study and practice. When we're emotionally triggered, we can perpetuate harm, repeating a past harm that was once inflicted upon us, or we can create a new energetic pattern of healing. It takes practice, not perfection.

The question to ask yourself is, *How can I find a way to feel, process, and release the energy of emotion that is moving through me in a way that is more healthy and less harmful to myself and those around me?* Here are two helpful reminders for when you are experiencing tough emotions:

This too shall pass. Many Persian Sufi poets, such as Rumi, wrote about this in the 1200s. We tend to think our uncomfortable emotions are going to last forever and that our favored emotions are going to slip away sooner than we wish. "This too shall pass" reminds us to be present and appreciate *what is,* while remembering that nothing will last forever. A new day—and a new moment—is on the horizon. Trust the process.

The only way out is through. Or, as Robert Frost wrote in his poem *A Servant to Servants* (1915), "the best way out is always through." On a stormy day, you might decide to stay in, make a cup of warm tea and reflect. Or maybe you'll dance in the rain or listen to the rain pitter-patter on your roof during a meditation. The storm will not "go away" faster because you want it to. Your work is to navigate who you are going to be and how you are going to respond, knowing that it will pass.

Bounce Back

One of the benefits of learning to NFPL your emotions is that you cultivate emotional resilience. Emotional resilience is your capacity to "bounce back" and transmute the energy of your emotions into heart-centered truth. I notice that as I learn to notice, feel, process, and let go, things that once resulted in a "bad week" start to become just a "bad day." And a "bad day" becomes a "bad hour." And a "bad hour" becomes "a bad few minutes." And a "bad few minutes" becomes *a deep breath,* a moment of discomfort followed by a moment of release.

The spiritual work starts to kick in when you realize that discomfort isn't "bad." It's just a part of the process. Don't get me wrong, I still have tough days sometimes, and there are periods of life that can be truly challenging. *Emotional resilience is your ability to fully feel and respond to your emotions in a way that honors your humanity and remembers your divinity.* As you become increasingly skilled at navigating your emotions, you get less stuck, and your bounce-back period gets shorter and shorter. You become more able to move through certain emotions with perhaps a little more ease, self-compassion, and spacious grace.

The Raw Truth of Grief

My friend, author, TV writer, and TED speaker Sarah Montana joined me once on "SoulFeed" to speak about grief. Sarah's mother and brother were murdered at gunpoint six days before Christmas during her senior year of college. It's taken her years to process such a sudden and tragic loss, and the way she speaks about grief, love, and forgiveness is a masterclass in emotional resilience. She shares how her mom and brother continue to show up in her life almost every day—in real, spiritual, and beautiful ways.

Sarah said in our interview, "Somebody can't be reborn to you until you let them die. Once I allowed myself to feel my suffering and not treat it as a bad thing, I learned that—even though it stings—suffering was the antidote to the wound and a pathway toward healing."

Grief can be one of the toughest things we experience, but experience it we must. It is the price of having loved so profoundly and deeply. In Sarah's words, "Grief is the most human experience you can have. We all experience birth and death, and love is what fills everything in between. If we've lived our lives right, we will have loved people so strongly and so fully that to lose them will be devastating."

Grief will happen—in one way or another. But that should never keep you from loving fully, wildly, and wholeheartedly. In fact, that should motivate you to love big. Amidst my own grief and heartbreak after a breakup with a beloved boyfriend, I wondered if the soreness would ever go away, that deep mental-physical-soul longing that seemed to be with me, day and night, for months. What I learned for myself and what I offer to you is this: *You can't rush your healing. Keep breathing. Keep going. Healing happens in stages, and grief sheds in layers—like an onion. Not in one fell swoop. Trust the process. Great loss is always the sign of the courageous capacity of your heart to love big.*

It can be both refreshing and painful to admit: the people you love will always be with you. When your soul touches another soul, they become a part of you, making up the whole of who you are. To grieve loss is to honor love. Grief is a beautiful—albeit painful— emotion because it brings you home to the raw truth of your heart.

TASTE THE RAINBOW

Obviously, not all emotions are tough, shadow emotions. But, even the "good" emotions can turn sour and stale if we attempt to cling to them by making them "stay." The light emotions are meant to be felt, processed, and released too.

Happiness is the favorable, acceptable emotion in our society, and yet, the American "pursuit of happiness" is so often the greatest cause of unhappiness. To pursue only one emotional experience while denying all the other colors of the emotional spectrum is the definition of living in delusion. Happiness *is* happiness as we know it because of our contextual experience of sadness. The contrast of both gives us rich appreciation for each.

In order to experience the truth of who we are, we must embrace— and not turn away from—the whole of our humanity. Think of how a baby can go from hysterically crying to delightfully laughing in a single instant. Babies have the ability to move through and feel their full emotional spectrum. As we become adults, we get stuck in the stories about our emotions, telling ourselves, "This emotion is good" (happiness, excitement, joy), and "This emotion is bad" (sadness, grief, despair).

Who decided this? No emotion is good or bad; it's just energy moving through. How we respond to our emotions via the thoughts we think, the words we speak, and the actions we take can be helpful or harmful. But the emotions themselves are just energies, needing the space to be felt.

Emotion is the proof of the presence of your spirit because every emotion is here to remind you of the full, whole, totality of who you are. The more skilled you become at embracing the wildness and wonder of your emotional capacity, the more compassion you'll cultivate for yourself—not the self that society wants you to be, but the self you were born to be.

"The Way" to Your Heart

It's your spiritual work to undo the toxic conditioning of society that shames us into believing "Men can't cry," or "Women are too emotional," or "Get over it already." These cultural "laws" cause us to disconnect from our hearts as a safe place to be and explore and *feel*. And the more we disconnect from our hearts, the more we disconnect from our own personal wisdom and truth.

Vietnamese Buddhist monk and peace activist Thich Nhat Hanh says, "There is no way to happiness. Happiness is the way" (*The Art of Mindful Living* audio program, 1992). Pursuing a specific emotion is like trying to catch a cloud. Whatever emotion arises, being with that emotion is "the way" home to your True Self. If sadness shows up, sadness is the way. If grief shows up, grief is the way. Rage is the way. Shame is the way. Your truest, most badass self awakens as you feel with your whole heart.

Cultivate a Courageous Heart

The emotions that repulse you when you see them in another person are the same emotions you've attempted to shut off within yourself. What you deny in another person, you deny within yourself. This is what is so toxic about "happiness culture." When happiness is the only acceptable emotion and we turn our backs on each other when we see someone sad, grieving, or having a hard time, we disconnect from the fullness of our humanity. We pretend there is only one appropriate way to be, and this form of emotional perfectionism numbs us from the truth of the full human experience.

Practicing the willingness to stay and feel the shadow emotions in yourself not only deepens your relationship with yourself, it deepens your capacity to be human. If you are willing to do the work—time and time again—of noticing your shadow emotions and then feeling, processing, and letting them go, you start to build your capacity to be with discomfort and pain. You turn toward—and not away from—your humanity.

Then, as a result, when someone else shows up with sadness, you have the capacity to look them in the eye and see their pain without turning away from it. Your heart has the emotional stamina to stay with them…to really notice the person in front of you, to feel empathy for them, and perhaps help this person on *their* path to process and let go. Compassion is cultivated through befriending the whole of who you are—all emotions and aspects of you. The shadow and the light. By filling yourself up with loving compassion, you inevitably have a wellspring of compassion to share with others—heart to heart.

In *The Wisdom of No Escape* (1991), Pema Chödrön shares the Buddhist practice of *tonglen*, which she invites us to practice with gentleness and precision. *Gentleness* is an attitude of loving kindness toward yourself—remembering your inherent goodness. *Precision* is an invitation to stay with the breath and bring the focus back to the breath when the mind wanders and gets distracted. But to always do so with gentleness.

Through the practice of tonglen, we are cultivating the *bodhicitta*, a courageous heart. Tonglen is a bold, brave practice because on the inhale, you invite yourself to feel the pain, the shadow, the grief, and the suffering of your own heart and the hearts of anyone in the world who's experiencing suffering. On the exhale, you extend love, compassion, loving kindness, peace, and ease out into the world. Through this practice, you cultivate the courage to be with both the shadow and light aspects of the heart—you are building your bodhicitta. You're transmuting pain into peace and suffering into ease and expanding your capacity to *be with both*. It takes a lot of courage to not turn our backs on our own suffering and the suffering of others, and practicing tonglen builds that courage. Pema says, "It's like watering a seed that can flower." All that is required is the tiniest seed of courage in your heart to begin to cultivate your bodhicitta, your courageous heart. There's something alchemical, even magical about this practice. On one breath in, you are present to pain, and on the next breath out, you are extending pleasure. On the breath in...discomfort, and on the next breath out...ease. Here's a challenge for you:

Set your timer for ten minutes and practice tonglen. If inspired, journal about your experience.

While it may be tempting to close and "protect" your heart amidst all the suffering in our world today, now is the time to stay open—to cultivate a courageous heart and to feel. In a society that has long diminished emotions as useless, your emotions are some of your greatest tools and signposts to understand your inner world. Let your heart open and lead you toward the person you are becoming. To remind you of who you already are. The courageous, openhearted ones are the ones who help bring us home to the truth.

EMOTIONAL INTELLIGENCE

When you practice feeling your feelings and expand your capacity for compassion, you build your emotional intelligence. According to *A Dictionary of Psychology* by Oxford University Press, emotional intelligence (EI) is the "capability of individuals to recognize their own emotions and those of others, discern between different feelings and label them appropriately, use emotional information to guide thinking and behavior, and manage and/or adjust emotions to adapt to environments or achieve one's goal(s)."

Social and Emotional Learning

There may be times when it seems like you can control your emotions and other times when it seems as if your emotions are controlling you. Emotions aren't enemies that need to be "controlled," but there are healthy and unhealthy ways to express emotion. Finding spaces to healthily express your feelings gives you a greater sense of power and groundedness as the electrical currents of emotion move through you.

On "SoulFeed," I had the honor of interviewing Scarlett Lewis, the founder of Jesse Lewis Choose Love Movement. Scarlett's six-year-old son Jesse was one of the twenty-six people who died at the Sandy Hook Elementary School school shooting in Newtown, Connecticut, in December 2012. In the wake of her son's death, Scarlett committed her life to bringing social and emotional learning (SEL) to schools and communities all over the world because research shows heavily substantiated evidence that social and emotional learning prevents violence by giving youth the ability to skillfully manage their mental and emotional health.

In our podcast interview, Scarlett said to me, "As human beings, we have a primal need for love. We *all* have a need to love and be loved. Love, this thing that connects all of us on this earth is a choice. And when we have some awareness, skills, and tools, we can choose love for ourselves and others." Scarlett believes wholeheartedly that the shooting that killed her son could have been prevented if the twenty-year-old shooter—a former student at Sandy Hook Elementary—had been taught emotional skills to process and manage his emotions and thoughts.

Scarlett also models to us the power of channeling and transmuting grief toward a greater purpose and a higher calling. She says that it took the death of her son to wake her up to her true purpose and calling. Now, she feels that her son Jesse is with her—guiding her to do the work of saving lives.

PUPPY MEDICINE

My second year living in Los Angeles, I was living by myself for the first time ever, had just been through a major breakup, and made a rather impulsive decision to adopt a puppy named Ginger, who was just three months old. I originally took her in as a foster, and as most puppies do, Ginger needed lots of attention and training. She's a smart, athletic dog, and it takes tons of exercise to tire her out. I quickly rose to the occasion of becoming the "Most Perfect Dog Dad Ever," which included multiple long walks every day, trips to the vet, organic food, socialization with other puppies, grooming, treats, toys, bones, and more treats. In our first few months together, Ginger traveled with me as an emotional support animal to Sedona, Arizona;

San Luis Obispo, California; and we even took a big cross-country trip on a plane to Gaithersburg, Maryland. On Mother's Day, I took her to be reunited with her mom—who also happened to be local in Los Angeles. #BestDogDadEver

When I transitioned from fostering her to officially adopting her, I was really torn about the decision, and I could feel the misalignment internally. I loved her with my *whole heart*. She was my baby girl. How could I *not* adopt her? But there was a nagging feeling in my gut that told me this was *way too much for me right now*. I was single, living alone for the first time, and finding my footing in my new city. I was totally overwhelmed, but I ignored my gut and adopted her anyway.

I quickly found myself incredibly frustrated and triggered when normal puppy things would happen...like peeing on the floor, vomiting on my new couch, and running away from me in the park. Sometimes, when Ginger was disobedient, the ugliest emotion trapped deep inside of my tissues would surface: rage. Ginger peed on my floor...again, and my fury escalated well-beyond a proper puppy scolding. I'd yell, burning with the fire of a thousand suns while this poor little pup cowered in the corner. And when I saw her sweet eyes were afraid of me, I felt such shame. Ginger, with her perfect innocence, was allowing me to see a side of myself and feel feelings lodged deep inside me that I had swept far under the rug of shame. I did *not* want to feel this. At the time, it felt very scary and unsafe, and I didn't know where it was coming from.

Digging Deeper Beneath the Surface

As I dug deeper, I was able to see how deeply I was dishonoring myself by taking responsibility for a puppy. I just wasn't ready—and the timing was off. I knew that the rage was a sign that I wasn't honoring my truth, but I told myself, *Shannon. People have dogs. Why can't you just get your shit together and take care of a dog like everyone else—without it being a big deal?* Shame.

Eventually, I had to sit with the truth of my experience so I could honor both Ginger and myself. I remember times where I actually felt jealous of the high level of care I was giving her. I remember thinking, *I want to take care of myself the way I am taking care of her.* Our emotions have the ability to reveal our deeper needs and desires to us. For me, this meant I needed to do a better job at parenting myself. I wasn't ready to be a single dad, and the resentment and rage that I was feeling toward Ginger was not healthy or aligned for either of us. I knew I could either (a) stay in it and learn to accept my choice and manage my emotions or (b) create a new circumstance for both of us to thrive.

Once I worked through the shame and feelings of failure, I was able to see that there was actually no right or wrong choice. There was only the best choice for Ginger and me. When I really sat soberly with that question, "Which choice is the best for us both?" I knew I had to let her go. And in my heart, I know this was one of the greatest acts of love I could've shown her—despite how difficult it was for me to accept. So, I made the tough, heart-wrenching, and necessary decision to find Ginger a new home. She now lives happily with a big family in Newport Beach, California, and I regularly get updates with pictures of my sweet girl.

Emotions are teachers—communications from your heart. They invite you to go through a process of transformation. If I didn't look at my rage with curiosity and a sense of knowing that my heart was communicating an important and essential message to my body and mind, I would've continued to harm both myself and Ginger. We don't always want to accept the transformational changes that our emotions propose we make. You don't need to take meaningful action in response to every single emotion you have, but when you have a repeated pattern of emotion—rearing its beautiful, ugly head—you know this is something that needs to be looked at.

Sacred Rage

In New York City, they say, "If you can make it here, you can make it anywhere." Similarly, if you can learn to wield and work with rage, you can apply the wisdom you learn to managing all other emotions. Rage is a wild, fiery, hot emotion. It's almost impossible to suppress (and can be harmful to try). It must be channeled and directed toward transformation and healing.

Rage can be a surefire sign that you're not honoring yourself and your truth. It may reveal to you that:

a) Somewhere in your life, you're not in alignment with your highest self and need to make a change,

b) Unprocessed trauma has been stored deep in the body and is desperately seeking release, or

c) Both.

For me, it was both. Ginger was my sacred little guru. She provided "puppy medicine" that revealed a wound to me that I was way too ashamed to address. This wound was begging for my attention and care, and Ginger helped me see the pattern—in a way that no human could. My rage was not just circumstantial; this wasn't about a puppy peeing on the floor. This rage felt familiar and historical. Like fights I would get into with my ex and my sister. Like smashing the glass windowpane and kicking the door when I was little. Like feeling so out-of-control growing up that the only way I knew how to cope and get the attention that I craved was to rage. *This wound was finally coming to a head—ready for the reckoning.*

Ginger helped me see the fire within me that was seeking to be released. Through having the courage to look deeper, I was able to see that yes, this rage was my responsibility to heal, but it was also much bigger than me and not mine alone to carry. This rage was intergenerational trauma being passed like a wild wire of toxic masculinity awaiting someone to wake up and learn to wield it, release it, and heal it. From my grandfather's rage to my dad's impatience and temper with me to my explosive outbursts with Ginger, I could suddenly see so clearly that by stepping into the role of father, I was called to heal the father wound of rage that was alive in me. Suddenly, no amount of social media or food or work or dating apps could distract me from reckoning with the heat. I couldn't blame my ex or play a victim. Ginger's spicy, sweet innocence and unconditional love helped me to see—and take responsibility for—my anger, overwhelm, perfectionism, impatience, and feeling out-of-control. Through NFPL (which I needed to repeat many times, by the way), I developed deep compassion for my dad, whose plate was so full just trying to take care of my family, as well as my grandfather, myself, and all people who've been told to carry the world on their shoulders, shut off from their emotional tenderness, and "hold it all together." My friends, for the sake of all of us, it's time to teach our boys how to feel. And that, of course, begins with *us*.

Rage Responsibly

Lashing out in rage can be very harmful and even dangerous, but suppressing rage can be equally harmful because it gets stored away, builds up, and guarantees future harm. To handle rage healthily, it must be wielded consciously like fire. Fire can safely light a candle, and it can grow to burn down hundreds of thousands of acres of land. When you see rage within yourself for what it is—a deep and desperate outcry for help, attention, love, and care—you can begin to parent yourself and wield this fire in ways that are nonharmful to yourself and those around you. Here are some healthy ways to release rage:

- Beat your mattress with a pillow.

- Scream at the top of your lungs, "Aaaaaaaaahhhh!!!!!!!"

- Do those at the same time!

- Kickbox, dance, run, sweat, move!

- Furiously journal your stream of consciousness. Write, write, write!

Once the energy of rage is released, you can process what it's all about. Ask yourself:

Where in my life might I be betraying myself or giving my power away?

Is this rage historical, situational, or both?

What needs to be released?

How can I release this rage without harming myself and others?

Then, transmute rage into a force for greater healing.

What is this rage teaching me about my passion and power?

What could I do with this energy if I weren't judging myself for having it?

What action can I take to integrate the wisdom of my rage?

While every situation is unique, here's a rage disclaimer: *when you are in the heat of rage, it may be appropriate to, first, do the work releasing, processing, and transmuting the rage within yourself and then, wait until you cool down to take an action that involves others.*

With great rage comes great responsibility. It can be destructive, but it can also blaze a trail toward healing. Become the steward of your rage without denying or suppressing it. Let it teach you how to move toward honoring yourself and your truth.

HEART'S DESIRES

"Listen with your heart, you will understand."

—Grandmother Willow from Disney's *Pocahontas*

Your heart is always beating—in the present moment. The heart's longings deserve to be felt, seen, heard, and known. Your job is to be a good listener. When you rinse old, stagnant emotions—the tough ones like grief, sadness, and rage—you clear the space in the heart so it can open up and lead the way. Your heart is your ally and your best friend. Anything is possible when your heart is "in it."

Your emotional power can be directed to amplify your desires and manifest your dharma. So, consider and reflect, what does your heart truly desire? For a Let Your Heart Lead meditation practice to drop into your heart before the following journaling exercise, go to http://www.trustyourtruthbook.com.

Write down everything your heart desires. But! Don't write from your head. Instead, write from your heart. A great way to stay connected to the heart is to stay connected to the breath while you write. Breathe into your heart and sense that your arm is a literal extension of the heart—pouring itself onto the page in the form of words. You can use these questions as prompts:

Who do you love and why?

What do you love about yourself?

What makes your heart soften and open?

What does it feel like to let your heart lead?

If you fully trusted your heart as a trusted leader in your life, where would it guide you?

In your heart of hearts, what does your soul crave that your mind may not be aware of yet?

What do you most desire?

As you build more of a trusting partnership with your heart, you can make decisions that honor your soul's truth. Your heart is a doorway into the sacred sanctuary space where your True Self resides. As we move into the next chakra, the throat chakra, we explore how the heart can find its voice through the vibration of sound and the words you choose to speak. How can you craft words to be in support of the desires of the heart and the mission of your dharma?

CHAPTER 5

Your Word Is Your Wand

Throat Chakra, *Vishuddha*

Color: Blue

Element: Sound/space/ether

Body: Throat, esophagus, tongue, teeth, lips, jaw, neck vertebrae

Emotional Impact: Opening up this energetic center to be a channel for truth speaking

Shadow: Lies

Light: Expression

Soul Truth: *My voice carries forth the vibration of my soul's truth.*

Mantra: *Ham* (Bringing the awareness to the throat center, repeat ham—sounds like "hum"—out loud or silently eight times before beginning to read this chapter. Sense the energy of space.)

As you become more confident in your purpose and you lead with your heart, your voice supports you to bring your truth out into the world. We don't want fear and doubt to prevent you from speaking your truth into existence. When I was in fifth grade, my mom took me and my sister Molly to see a local musical theater performance. My mom still talks about the twinkle she saw in my eye during the show. (It's true, I was lit up!) I was mesmerized by how the kids on the stage were singing, dancing, and *having so much fun.* To my eleven-year-old self, this might as well have been a Broadway show. As we were leaving, I said, "Mom, I want to do that!"

That summer, she enrolled me in the summer camp at the Musical Theater Center (MTC), the same organization that produced the show we saw. I was excited and terrified. I also auditioned for their big summer production of *Joseph and the Amazing Technicolor Dreamcoat.* And I got in!

After being in so many different situations in life that gave me anxiety because I rarely felt like I belonged or that I was good enough, stepping into the theater world felt like I was finally home. In school, I was often taunted for sitting at the "girls' table" at lunch instead of with the boys. I was considered "weird" for wanting to sit with my girl friends. But at MTC, everyone was together. Singing together. Dancing together. Rehearsing together. Backstage together. Onstage together. Hugging, loving, celebrating, and being themselves. *I was in love with theater. Officially obsessed.*

But even with all of the acceptance in this new environment, it took me months—and even years—to embrace being seen and heard. My body held so much fear, shame, and anxiety from all those coping mechanisms I used to feel safe and protected that I was too afraid to sing out loud and dance freely. In anticipation of being bullied or judged by the director, choreographer, or God forbid, my new friends, I'd hide and play small. I'd do anything to keep myself from being targeted and teased. My jaw would lock up during my solo for a big number, and my body would tense when it was time to let go and dance. I still remember the sensation of my tongue tensing in the back of my throat—a physical manifestation of the fear of speaking up and being heard.

But "the show must go on." By stepping into the spotlight and being required to dance big, have fun, and sing out, I slowly and unknowingly retrained my nervous system to become comfortable putting myself out there. This was pivotal and transformative to counteract years of shame, and bullying, and playing small. At the time, I had no clue that stepping onto the stage would be so healing for the part of me that didn't believe I deserved to be seen, felt, and heard.

We all have an innate need and desire for our voices to be heard and our true selves to be known. "Hold your tongue," and "Children are to be seen and not heard," are archaic expressions that reveal how we've been trained for generations to be small and silent. You may have felt (or feel) discouraged from speaking up while emotional, punished for calling out the elephant in the room, or even shamed for getting too excited when celebrating. This totally sucks. But the great news is, you can confront these oppressive messages—and let your voice be heard now. It's time to "Sing out, Louise!"

We all have an innate need and desire for our voices to be heard and our true selves to be known.

♡

Reflect and write in your journal:

1. Does an experience come to mind where you were silenced and learned to "shut up"? *Notice if there's a specific experience that stands out. Go with your first gut response.*

2. What was the physical impact of this experience on your body? *Perhaps you remember stomach pains or sweating profusely before giving a speech or presentation.*

3. What message did you receive—what belief did you internalize—about yourself? *Maybe you came to the conclusion, "I'm terrible at _____."*

4. In what ways has this experience (or experiences similar to it) affected the way you show up in the world today? *Notice if there're any decisions you made about what experiences you will or will not allow yourself to have—about what you "can" and "cannot" say or do.*

It may be momentarily uncomfortable to bring this up to the surface, but it's truly transformative to consciously see these internalized messages for what they are—pivotal moments that deserve to be acknowledged but no longer need to control the way you live your life and use your voice. They say F.E.A.R. either stands for *fuck everything and run* or *face everything and rise.* Kudos to you for your courage to rise.

OPEN THE CHANNEL TO YOUR VOICE

The breath is the vehicle that carries the sound of your voice through you, so it's essential to become aware of it when preparing your voice to be expressive, resonant, and heard. It's common to hold the breath and lock the jaw in an attempt to stop emotions from moving from the fourth chakra, the heart, to the fifth chakra, the throat. To become fully self-expressed, start by noticing your breathing. Become aware of the moments when you unconsciously hold your breath. When you hold the breath, you hold back the expression of life moving through your vessel. Of course, you don't need to speak up about every feeling that you have or thought that you think—but you *do* need to breathe. Breathing is the only involuntary, automatic function of the body that can also be voluntary. To become conscious of your breath is to become conscious of your ability to bring your deep, unseen truth into the world in a clear way—through the vessel of your voice.

Breath is the first thing we all take when we arrive on this planet after the umbilical cord is cut, and it's the last thing we'll all release when we leave our bodies. Right now, as you're reading, notice your inhalation and notice your exhalation. As the breath comes into the body, notice the body's capacity to receive the breath. As the breath leaves the body, notice the body's capacity to release the breath. Can you become aware that you are not "doing" the breathing, but rather, the breath is moving in and out naturally on your behalf?

Whenever you want to speak your truth, first, take a deep inhale. And then allow the words to flow out with your exhale. Sometimes you may find yourself "speaking on empty" with no breath to support you. We often hold our breath and clench our throats to mask and suppress our true emotions. It can be vulnerable—and brave—to reveal your true emotions and to speak truth.

Check in with your relationship with your breath. Ask yourself these questions as you move through the next week. Become aware of the moments when you hold your breath.

- *What is the relationship between my speech and my breath?*

- *Am I inhaling before I speak and then speaking as I exhale?*

- *Am I holding my breath and speaking on an empty tank?*

- *How do people respond differently when I breathe as I speak?*

Of course, you may not want to speak your truth in every single moment of your life, but if you stay connected to your breath, you'll stay connected to your truth. And when you do choose to speak, your energy will have more of an impact as your breath carries your words through your body and out into the world. Continue to notice your body breathing as you move throughout your day because an honest conscious breath is always a direct insight into how you are truly feeling.

YOU BETTA SANG!

Each of us has a voice, and just as the songbird needs to sing, you are born with a desire to find your voice to speak truth in your life. The throat chakra, Vishuddha, is the energetic center where you discover the power of your voice.

Think about it for a sec: The throat is directly between your mind and heart. Language is formed in the mind, emotions emerge in the heart, and your voice is the energy center where these two worlds come together, to meet and merge as one.

Singing, or chanting, is incredibly medicinal and healing because it can quickly counteract years of being silenced. For me, I needed to have the physical, embodied experience of vocal freedom through singing so I could understand the difference between swallowing my words and having true, vocal freedom.

The most common thing that stops people from singing is the belief that they can't do it. I can tell you with 100 percent assuredness, you *can* sing. But a belief that you can't sing will be 99.9 percent effective at stopping you. Whether or not other people *enjoy your singing* is completely irrelevant to *your capacity to sing.*

Your voice is an instrument. And using your voice is instrumental to healing yourself and those around you. Consider this: Imagine you aren't the one who does the singing. Instead, imagine sound effortlessly moves through you—like wind flowing through a tunnel. Imagine your body is a bamboo flute, and the flow of life is the cosmic breath that moves sound through the vessel of your body. All you have to do is open your channel and allow the energy of sound to flow. My Yoga Nidra teacher Tracee Stanley, author of *Radiant Rest* (2021), says, "When you recognize truth, truth has a vibration. The more you practice, the more you attune yourself to the vibration of truth." Here's a sound vibration you can use to attune yourself to the vibration of truth—right now.

Fraulein Maria, played by Julie Andrews in *The Sound of Music*, is back for a quick singing lesson. But instead of the typical "Do-Re-Me," we're going to use the ancient, sacred, unifying sound of the Universe, "Om." You may have heard it at the beginning or end of a yoga class.

Om, sometimes spelled AUM, represents the four states of consciousness:

1. "A" represents the waking state of consciousness—the alert, thinking mind.

2. "U" represents the dreaming state of consciousness—the energy body.

3. "M" represents the deep sleeping state of consciousness—the wisdom of the heart.

4. The silence after the AUM is known as "the fourth state of consciousness" or the void. In the stillness of the fourth state of consciousness, we return to Source—the space of egoless nothingness where all things are experienced as whole and one.

In this chanting exercise, it doesn't matter what your mind thinks about how you sound. What matters most is your ability to sense the sound moving through your energy system.

So, the invitation now is to take a deep breath and chant AUM three times in a row with your eyes closed. Feel each of the four phases of sound, taking your time with each one so you can experience the:

1. Aaaahhh (waking). Feel this sound resonate in your head.

2. Uuuuuuu (dreaming). Feel this sound resonate in your throat and chest.

3. Mmmmmm (deep sleep). Feel this sound resonate in your heart.

4. :::silence::: (the void). Feel the spacious stillness of nothingness.

Can you notice the juxtaposition between sound filling your body and space compared to the moment of nothingness afterward? This contrast between sound followed by silence allows for a moment of stillness and deep peace. In the pause, notice if you feel the vibration of truth. You may find that you are momentarily able to access Source within you. Enjoy the silence of the void for a few moments, and bask in the vibration of truth. This practice is one you can use every day to open the channel of your voice, move energy, create a sacred space, and connect to your truth.

THE SOURCE OF YOUR SOUND

The quality and tone of your voice hold an energetic vibration that has the power to touch, move, and inspire the energies of those around you. Begin to notice from what space within yourself this energy is emerging. In my interview with Rha Goddess, author of *The*

Calling (2020), she posed the question, "Where is this sourced from?" Are your words sourced from love, possibility, joy, collaboration, and spirit? Or are your words sourced from fear, cynicism, judgment, and resignation? What is trying to find expression through you? When you speak, observe the space within yourself from which you are speaking. Is it your mind? Your body? Your heart? Your sex organs? All of the above?!

For example, I can usually tell when I am talking from my mind as I notice I am analyzing, starting sentences with "I think," weighing pros and cons, strategizing, and maybe even controlling, manipulating, and obsessing. Notice if the mind is the dominant aspect of yourself that is given a voice. This is common in our Western culture, which rewards productivity and results.

You can also tell when you are speaking from the heart. When I am speaking from my heart, I notice I can identify the emotions I'm feeling, start sentences with "I feel," place my hand on my heart, and am aware of my emotions. The invitation is to allow your voice to express the deeper desires and wishes of your heart and notice how you are able to speak from your heart.

When you are speaking from the body, you may notice you are referencing certain physical sensations you feel or starting sentences with "I need," speaking from a place of concern about earthly needs such as food, clothing, or shelter, or you may even be speaking from a place of fear of survival. Have you ever been "hangry"? You know, hungry and angry? When I'm hangry, I'm definitely speaking from the body!

It's possible you are speaking from multiple, and even conflicting, spaces within yourself—at the same time. As you speak, this process of noticing *where you are speaking from* can be incredibly illuminating. There's no right or wrong here, but by becoming aware, you can consciously reclaim the full power of your voice.

As you speak, you can begin to notice and ask yourself, *From what space within myself am I speaking?* Simultaneously, notice your breath, which will help guide you home to your truth.

You can also pay attention to where others are speaking from. Try to do this without judgment, and also be sure to ask yourself, *From what space within myself am I listening?*

ALIGN WITH YOUR INTEGRITY

The word "integrity" comes from the Latin root "integer," which means intact, and the *Oxford English Dictionary* definition of integrity is, "the state of being whole and undivided." To be "in integrity" is to be in alignment. As Harvard Business School professor and economist Michael C. Jensen says in an academic paper, "Integrity. Without it, nothing works."

You can use your words to lift up—instead of diminish—the truth of who you are by ensuring your words are "in integrity" with your True Self. Check in with yourself: *Are my words in alignment with my heart's desires?* When you speak words that are out of alignment with your True Self, you are out of integrity, and you'll likely experience some kind of inner conflict or suffering. This suffering is not a punishment, and you haven't done anything "wrong." You're just out of alignment, and the inner conflict helps wake you up so you'll listen to what needs to be done for you to get back into alignment. Your soul wants you to wake up and be in integrity with your highest self.

In yoga, each posture has integrity, and you can feel when you're in proper alignment because the body can feel a sense of being whole. In Warrior 2 pose, for example, the front leg is bent and the back leg is straight. When aligned, the bent front knee is stacked directly over the ankle of the front foot. If the knee passes the ankle and moves forward over the toes, too much pressure is put on the knee, which could cause discomfort in the knee joint—even a painful injury over time. See how just a slight misalignment causes trouble? When in alignment, the knee receives the support of the shin bones, as well as the ankle, foot, and floor beneath you.

When the bones are stacked just right, in alignment, energy flows more freely through the pose. It actually makes the pose feel easier and more sustainable because the body relies less on muscle to "hold" the pose and instead harnesses the strength of the bones so you can *experience* the pose in a more relaxed way. Instead of getting bogged down by unnecessary knee pain, you can focus more on the breath and the engagement of the hips and core. The integrity of the whole pose increases its overall vibrancy and power. And, the more you practice Warrior 2, the easier the alignment becomes.

The same thing happens when you're living in alignment with your truth. Whenever you bring yourself into internal alignment, you save yourself from muscling through life trying to fit a round peg into a square hole, and instead, you can *experience the benefits* of being in integrity with your soul. Your relationships, your actions, your heart, your *why*, and your words work together to serve your commitment to be the true you. Life actually feels easier when you are aligned internally because your energy is supported and flowing freely.

When it comes to using your words, integrity means you do what you say you are going to do. Your actions align with your words. Here's how to get aligned, have integrity, and build confidence: When you speak from your heart and give your word of commitment to something, ensure that you actually show up and take action. If you do this, you instantly become a person you can count on and who other people can count on too. Perhaps one of the most joyfully surprising benefits of being in integrity with your whole self is the confidence that blossoms from knowing you are a badass who is committed to following through. I know for me, nothing has built up my confidence faster than doing the shit I say I am going to do. As a bonus, it's built up other people's confidence in me too. Integrity works if you work it.

If you need to change your agreement to yourself or someone else, that's totally okay, just be sure to get into communication and change your commitment. Words matter because *you* matter.

WORDS MATTER

Your words have the capacity to wield so much energy that they can influence and create physical matter. I'll never forget when I attended the Landmark Forum in my twenties, our leader and coach Angie Mattingly said to us, "You're going to be *so* in integrity with your word that when you say chair, a chair is going to fall out of your mouth." Imagine being so aligned, clear, and powerful that you could say a word and presto! It instantly manifested. Thankfully, there's a bit of a time delay, which gives us time to rethink and reorganize. But when she said that, I thought to myself, *Damn! Yes, I want that!* If you want to move toward a particular goal, you can bring the energy of that goal to life using language.

You actually have the power to speak things into existence! As spiritual teacher and author Marianne Williamson says, "An idea grows stronger when it is shared." So as you speak, you energize a thought or feeling into a vibration that is heard and felt beyond you. The words you choose to give life to have the power to shape your reality—as well as reveal deep insights into what and how you are thinking and feeling. You can speak truth—or delusion—into existence. Your word is your wand!

Thinking a thought is one thing, and we'll talk about the power of the mind in the next chapter, but speaking a thought is a creative act of bringing forth energy that has never before existed into the physical world through your vibration. Your words create a force of real energy. Every word has a color, texture, purpose, and life. Here are some words that really seem to embody the energy of their meaning. Notice how you feel as you read them.

- Moist (I know...a controversial one!)

- Buoyant

- Luscious

- Sweet

- Morbid

- Suction

- Freedom

- Thwart

- Celebration

- Morose

Can you feel the energy in each of these words? Similarly feel into the words you use, whether internally or out loud. Let's do an inventory of words in your vocabulary that are disempowering you. *It's time to "Marie Kondo" that shit!* Marie Kondo is the celebrated Japanese creator of the KonMari method of organizing stuff. It's a practice of evaluating each item you own and asking yourself the simple question, *Does it spark joy?* Then you let go of things you're keeping in your environment that do not spark joy. Let's do this with the words you are using that might be "cluttering" inside of you. It may be time to *let that shit go.*

Here's an example of a word that I noticed I was using that was diminishing the power of my speech. The subtle yet lethal word "just."

"I'm just *reaching out to see if you are available to meet in person.*"

"I'm just *checking in to see if you'd be interested in coming on my podcast.*"

"I just *thought that it was okay with you.*"

As I became conscious of myself using this word, I noticed that I had been unconsciously using the word "just" to make myself sound more passive, less intense, and less threatening. In doing so, I was repeating my codependent pattern of concerning myself with how *someone else would think of me* rather than *truthfully speaking my intention with clarity and purpose.*

Reread these sentences without the *just.*

"I'm reaching out to see if you are available to meet in person."

"I'd love for you to be a guest on my podcast."

"I genuinely believed it was okay with you."

Can you feel the difference? I could feel the shift in my body when I removed "just" from my vocabulary. I still use it sometimes, just now I'm more conscious. When I choose to use language that is clear, straightforward, and direct, my confidence automatically gets boosted because I can feel the direct impact in my body. My intentions are sent (and mostly received) with 100 percent certainty when I practice eliminating the crumbs of doubt from my speech. Even if I don't get the response that I want from the other person, I can feel the confidence in my own self, first and foremost.

It's likely some words in your vocabulary diminish your power in some way—hide your truth. Become aware of the words you speak so you can be an effective creator of your life. Words are insights into your beliefs. Notice in the next day or so (and throughout the rest of your life!): *What words need to be reckoned with?* You might hear a certain word come out of your mouth and it feels "wrong." You may feel your body losing energy when you speak a word that is not aligned with your truth.

The practice is to observe and notice as these words arise when you're out in the world living your life. If you catch yourself using a word that is stripping you of your wholeness, take note of that word and write it down. Keep a running list of words that do not spark joy. Instead of beating yourself up for speaking a disempowering word, ask yourself,

What does an empowering alternative to this word look, sound, and feel like?

How can I say this in a more proactive, positive, and clear way?

Become aware of how the use of the new word feels in your body. Make a commitment to integrate this new language in your life. Start practicing. New lingo, new you!

To take this to the next level, go back to your *why statement—* your dharma code—from chapter 3 and review your heart's desires from chapter 4. *How can you wield your words to speak your dharma into existence—to bring your purpose and your heart out into the world in a more powerful way?* What you speak repeatedly with conviction gains momentum and strength, so notice which words you may be using that are energizing your dharma and which words are diminishing it. You may want to have a meaningful conversation with a friend, therapist, or mentor. You might create a post on social media or write a song or perhaps a book. Ask yourself, *How can I use my words and my voice to bring my dharma and my heart to life in a more powerful, potent way?*

DIRECT YOUR ENERGY

When you are stuck in the muck of feeling negative, "off," or in a shitty mood, it's sometimes necessary to complain, vent, and process. Journal till your fingers ache. See a therapist. Call a trusted friend who is available to be there for you in that moment.

It's helpful to have boundaries around your venting. When we vent, it's sometimes easier to get stuck noticing *what's not working,* and it's more challenging to identify *what we really want.* It may do more harm than good to tell *all* your friends and spout the same story again and again. There's a threshold that gets crossed from *productive processing*, which feels good and helps you reach resolution, to *repetitive ranting*, which keeps you spinning on a hamster wheel of suffering. There's a difference, and as you notice it, you can feel if you cross that threshold.

Remember, your word is your wand. When you are speaking the same belief over and over and over again, it's going to become more real for you. Here's a great tool to use when you decide that it's time to move on from your productive processing and don't want to indulge in a repetitive rant. Simply say to yourself, "Thus far, no further." Seane Corn shared this with me—a practice that her teacher, the late Mona Miller, author of *Invisible Warfare* (2006), shared with her. When the time comes to put a cap on your grievances, you can say enough is enough with *"Thus far, no further."* It's a line in the sand. A boundary to benefit your True Self. After you've talked, ranted, cried, grieved, yelled, and screamed at the whole freaking planet, there will come a moment when you can say to yourself, *"Okay, sweetheart. That's enough. It's time to get going, and it's time to move forward."*

Only you can decide for yourself when you're ready for that moment. It's not anyone else's job to tell you when to set this boundary with yourself. Explore and discover what feels true, appropriate, and kind for you.

After you have drawn the boundary with your venting, as soon as you are ready, use your words as building blocks to create a new experience for yourself. Think of this as casting a spell! Your words can be the springboard out of the old and into the new. Anytime you find yourself stuck in a web of words that are not serving you, ask yourself and write the answers to these three questions in your journal:

1. *What do I really want?*

2. *What does the ideal solution look like?*

3. *How can I use my words to articulate, name, and spell out the energy of the solution?*

Voila! Your words, and the vibration with which you speak them, have the power to direct your energy. So direct them away from what you *don't* want and toward what you *do* want. All words begin as thoughts, so in the next chapter, we'll go deeper into some powerful tools to shift and direct your energy using the power of the mind.

LISTEN TO YOUR VOICE

Sometimes we stay silent because we fear "It'll come out wrong," or "I'll sound stupid," or "I'm not a very good speaker." Speaking truth takes courage, so I want to share with you exactly how I've built confidence in my voice.

When I launched my podcast "SoulFeed," thanks to a combination of luck, hard work, passion, and privilege, my cohost and I instantly landed interviews with some of the most influential spiritual and world leaders of our time. I remember when I listened back to those first interviews at the time, I was mortified. As I heard myself speak, I felt a warm wash of shame…no, a HOT wash of shame come over my body. I was literally sweating. I wanted to run and hide. I thought to myself, *Make it stop! I can't listen any longer. YOU SUCK.*

After that doubt attack, I became so self-conscious while recording solo episodes that, sometimes in the midst of them, I'd stop myself and start the entire episode over. Many times! It would take me four hours to record a twenty-minute episode. I was so judgmental of my voice, and I was almost never satisfied.

As time went on, the discomfort slightly dwindled because I *had* to listen to myself speak while editing my own episodes, and I started to get used to hearing myself. One day, while editing an interview with Gabby Bernstein, I noticed I was only a little hot and cringe-y! *Progress.* I heard myself articulating a thought then asking a question, and I genuinely thought to myself, *Okay, Shannon! You sound great! Clear, confident, and concise. Yaaas! Do more of that.* This may have been the first time since we started the podcast that I actually took a moment to compliment and feel good about myself.

It's important to note I didn't *feel* confident in the moment I spoke those words—instead, I felt clouded with self-doubt; I was judging myself and wondering if I was any "good." But by listening back and hearing that I sounded way better than I thought I did, I got the chance to realize, *Wait a second.... This sounds really great! Next time you're speaking about X, remember how much you're nailing this right now! Trust yourself and go for it!*

So, I offer this to you! Instead of judging your communication skills or your voice as either completely *terrific* or completely *terrible*, give yourself constructive feedback so you can learn and improve, and give yourself positive feedback when you do something great!

Now, I (mostly) enjoy listening to older episodes and hearing myself speak. I feel proud of myself because I can hear the improvements I've made. While little things here or there emerge that don't sound as powerful as they maybe could, I don't beat myself up over it. And I certainly don't throw away perfectly good episodes because I'm trying to be "perfect." I just take the constructive note and move forward with the intention to improve for the next one. Onward!

Speaking is a practice. Just like yoga, painting, meditation, or any learned skill. And the more you practice using your voice, the more skilled you become at the artform of speaking. So, here's a fun and possibly uncomfortable exercise that will give you the chance to practice.

SPEAK YOUR TRUTH AND LISTEN BACK

I want you to record yourself speaking. Before you slam this book shut and throw it across the room, hear me out. This is the exact formula I use to put together a solo podcast episode. It's pretty simple, actually, and I invite you to take on this challenge so you can learn to love yourself (and possibly your voice!!) through the process. Think of this as an experiment—to see what comes up and learn ways to more fully speak your truth. If you feel resistant, then this may well be the perfect exercise for you.

1. *Topic.* Pick a topic you feel passionate about—something you feel excited to speak on. (I'll use relationships as a sample topic.)

2. *Title.* Create a title for the theme of your topic (like "How to Fall in Love").

3. *Content.* Write out three to five bullet points that speak directly to this theme. Choose discussion points that you feel excited to talk about. For example, when speaking about how to fall in love, I'd write the following:

   a. Make a list of what you want in a relationship.

   b. Make a list of what you don't want in a relationship.

   c. Practice saying no when what you don't want shows up in your life.

   d. Go on a date committed to being your True Self.

   e. Fall in love with yourself—on repeat.

4. *Intro and Outro.* Give a little thirty- to sixty-second introduction of your theme at the beginning. You can answer these questions: *Why is this theme important to me? Why am I excited to share it?* After you go through all your points, give a little wrap-up summary and say good-bye.

5. *Record.* It's showtime! Get out your phone. Hit record. And flow. Remember to breathe and have fun.

6. *Take a break.* Don't listen to yourself right away. Step away for a few hours. This will allow you to be a little bit more objective for step 7.

7. *Listen back.* Create a sacred, quiet space for you to listen to your recording. Maybe burn some sage or light a candle. As you listen, breathe, breathe, breathe. Notice how the body feels. Notice any emotions that arise. Notice what the mind has to say.

8. *Write.* Now, journal about your experience. Write about how you felt while listening. Write three specific qualities you liked about your speaking. Write three specific notes of constructive feedback. *Don't write what you "didn't like." Instead, write what you can improve upon next time.*

If you're like me and the shame "gremlins," as Dr. Brené Brown calls them, come out to play when you think about listening back to the recording, this exercise could be incredibly powerful for you! I say, "Do it!" Don't get me wrong.... I've been there, and I know it's not always easy *at first.* But the reward of learning to skillfully use your voice to be a powerful communicator of your truth is well-worth the temporary discomfort. You've got this!

Now, let's look deeper into why some disempowering words might be harder to let go of. In the next chapter, you're going to lift up the hood of your own mind so you can see the roots of why you think and believe the way you do, align your mind with the truth, and let go of fear-based thinking and misperception.

CHAPTER 6

20/20 Vision

Third Eye Chakra, *Ajna*

Color: Indigo

Element: Light

Body: Center of the eyebrows, pituitary gland, eyes, eyesight, brow, brain, skull

Emotional Impact: Willingness to see truth and dissolve delusion

Shadow: Illusion

Light: Truth

Soul Truth: *I see the truth of this present moment.*

Mantra: *Om* (Bringing the awareness to the space between the eyebrows, repeat om—sounds like "home"—out loud or silently eight times before beginning to read this chapter. Sense the energy of light.)

The human mind is an incredibly powerful place—sometimes a generator of awe-inspiring creativity and other times, a terrifying war zone of judgment and conflict. It has the ability to build and destroy, create heaven and hell, generate love and perpetuate fear. It can bring us together and divide us apart. It can build a city up, and it can tear it down.

Just as teeth need to be flossed and muscles need to be strengthened, the mind needs to be tended to so it can see the truth—so it doesn't get lost in clouds of confusion and misperception. By tending to the garden of your own mind, you can discern which seeds you want to plant and which weeds you want to whack. You can actually be "in choice" about which thoughts you water and grow as well as those that you want to purge and let go. The mind is a great tool when it's in the service of your heart's wisdom. But it needs guidance, training, and ongoing support to navigate from being lost in delusion to arriving home at truth. As you dive into the power of your mind, remember to breathe into your heart space and include the heart in on this conversation. See if you can let your heart drive the car and let your mind be a helpful passenger.

It's essential to free your mind from limiting narratives so it can get into an empowered state of possibility and clarity. In this chapter, we'll go through a purification process that takes you to the root of your limiting beliefs so you can release their grip on your life and dissolve delusional thinking. By harnessing the powers of your heart, voice, and mind together as one team, you activate a new mental narrative—one that is rooted in truth and power. So, get ready. This chapter is the Magic School Bus, I'm Mrs. Frizzle, and we're about to go deep into the power of your mind! I promise we'll come out on the other side with a transformed perspective.

Let's begin with a short meditation to open the mind and illuminate your ability to direct its focus:

Imagine a light in the center of your brain—a healing light energy. Imagine this light could illuminate all perceptions, thoughts, beliefs, and neural pathways that live inside the brain. As the light begins to grow from within, imagine more of the corners and crevices of the mind beginning to receive the warmth of this light. Take a moment to breathe and feel this light growing in your mind— sensing the nonconscious areas of the mind beginning to come to the light of your awareness.

Now, bring your awareness to your third eye center, the space between your eyebrows. Imagine a beam of light shining from your third eye center and projecting outward into the whole room. Notice if you can feel any sensation or energy vibrating around your third eye center. Close your eyes and take three conscious breaths—inhaling to fill your mind with light, exhaling to send a light beam of energy out through your third eye center, and illuminating the surrounding space.

Welcome back. This meditation is a gentle reminder that you have the ability to direct your awareness and attention. As we move into the work of the mind, remember that there are infinite ways to perceive and experience reality. This chapter is for you to clarify what is most true for *you*.

PERCEIVING THE MOVIE OF YOUR MIND

The beliefs you hold about yourself and the world get projected outward, which you see as the movie screen of your life. You experience this projection as your reality, but you aren't the movie; you're the one who watches the movie! While you aren't solely responsible for everything that happens in your movie, you *are* responsible for how you perceive and process what occurs on your screen. When you can step back from the content and watch this movie, as an observer, you become able to ask these essential questions: *What lessons am I taking away from this experience? How is this experience shaping my beliefs? How do I want to look at this situation? What story will I choose to tell?*

The thing is, most of us don't realize we have the ability to shift our perception and change our point of view. We get stuck in a mind trap. In her book *Getting Unstuck* (2005), Pema Chödrön teaches about freeing ourselves from a stuck, "fixed mind." Fixed mind occurs when the mind hardens and solidifies around a certain reality: *this is the way it is—and under no circumstances is it any other way.* When you look at any aspect of your life with fixed mind, all other possibilities are squelched. Whatever you are looking at becomes so fixed that you become fixed along with it. And it can seem like there is absolutely no alternative way to see the situation. Fixed mind traps us into the experience of perceived certainty, which human beings tend to crave because it makes us feel safe. When you walk past a tree, do you really see the tree? Or do you see your assumptions about the tree—perhaps overlooking it or comparing it to other trees? We tend to see the past, and we're not fully present in the "now-ness" of this moment. But the soul thirsts for the opportunity to see things *as they really are,* not as we think they are or want them to be.

The exciting truth is *no thing is fixed.* Nothing! A wooden chair may appear to be a "just a chair." But it's actually vibrating with energy. And the wood that was carved to become the chair was once a tree that was once rooted in the earth. Freedom from fixed mind gives you access to curiosity, exploration, discovery, and creativity so you can open your mind, see things in new and different ways, and perhaps, create a new narrative for your life.

There are millions of ways to perceive any moment of your life—should you be open to such an adventure. "Knock, and it shall be opened unto you," as is said in Matthew 7:7 in the New Testament of the Bible. No matter how stuck you believe you are, a doorway in your mind can open up to a whole new realm of possibility. This might show up as a big aha moment, as a loud thud of disappointment, as an inspired idea, as clarity in a yoga or meditation practice, as the breakup of a relationship, or in a moment of divine intervention. When a doorway opens up in your mind to perceive something in a new light, only you can choose to walk through and explore what awaits you on the other side.

When the limiting beliefs we have about ourselves and what we're capable of feel "normal," we sometimes choose to stay fixed and committed to the very thing that causes our suffering. Asking yourself *quality questions* can create a miraculous shift in perception within your own mind.

MIRACLE QUESTIONS

The mind seeks to find answers to the questions you are asking it, and because of this, if you want to pivot from fixed mind to an open one, you want to practice asking yourself higher quality questions. When you ask yourself a question, your attention gets pinged in a very specific direction—and your mind consciously or unconsciously seeks to find the answer to that exact question...almost obsessively! Every question you ask yourself has the power to completely alter the course and direction of your life.

From working with clients (and on myself), I've noticed that when you hold a negative belief about yourself, the mind generates questions that keep you stuck in a disempowering loop, a self-fulfilling prophecy.

> Every question you
> ask yourself has the
> power to completely
> alter the course of
> your life.
>
> ♡

Questions that keep you stuck in the disempowering shame loop are:

What is wrong with me?

Why do I keep doing this?

Why am I so stuck?

Why can't I figure this out?

Be conscious of the questions you ask because the mind seeks to find answers! Noticing the disempowering question interrupts the pattern of negative thinking. Check in throughout your day, "What question am I asking myself right now?" When you feel stuck in an awful movie and there's no way out, think of this as changing the channel—switching the content of the movie on your screen.

A Course in Miracles teaches that a miracle is a shift in your perception from the thought-system of fear to the thought-system of love. By practicing miracle-mindedness, you can shift more readily from fear/scarcity to love/abundance. A miracle-shift occurs when your mind is able to see something differently—through the eyes of love instead of fear. The *Course* teaches that in order to invoke a miracle, all that is required is your willingness. When you ask for a miracle, you are saying, "Show me a better way. I acknowledge that the way that I am seeing this is not working. Please, may I see this differently."

Ask yourself, *How may I see this differently?* When you are humble enough to ask the Universe for support so that you can *see* your life through the lens of truth and love, the Universe can answer your call. Your call cannot be answered if you don't pick up the phone and dial.

One of my favorite things to do is to write a question in my journal and let my mind free-write all the answers until it is empty of all possible thoughts, answers, and solutions.

Some of my favorite questions to ask in my journal are:

What do I really want?

What does my ideal outcome for the situation look like?

What am I grateful for?

What would make today amazing?

What do I love about myself?

If one million dollars were directly deposited into my account today, what would I do with it?

Who am I, really?

The questions we ask ourselves contain the power to not only shift the direction of our minds, but to shift the direction of our lives. When we ask new and more empowering questions that invoke the deeper wisdom, we course-correct and bring ourselves onto the path that we are meant to be on. Because our minds tend to automatically populate disempowering questions based on past beliefs, we want to go deeper into the roots of our beliefs to reckon with any pesky weeds that need to be lovingly whacked.

GETTING TO THE ROOTS

Beliefs have a ripple effect through your whole body and being. They influence your thoughts, words, feelings, actions, relationships, the way you show up in the world, and perhaps most importantly, how you feel about yourself.

Soul-crushing negative beliefs can feel like they are eating at the fabric of who we are—fueling our self-doubt and spinning us into a spiral of shame and unworthiness. When we reality-check the thoughts swimming in our own minds, we notice some awful, terrible commentary. *How do we make it stop?*

Slapping a positive affirmation on top of a deep-seated negative belief about yourself is as effective as sprinkling glitter on top of a pile of shit to clean it up. It may look pretty, but in truth, it's *pretty shitty*. When you're dealing with a deeply rooted belief, adopting a "just be more positive" mind-set isn't enough to reckon with and heal that part of you that *believes* that disempowering narrative. You may have to clean up some shit in your mind, but once you do this work, you won't even need the glitter because you'll just sparkle as your own badass self!

Your experience of self-doubt is reinforced by a set of deeply held negative beliefs about yourself. Of course, it's not your fault for acquiring these negative beliefs—but you now get the opportunity to do some healthy excavation and Marie Kondo–style "Does this spark joy?" inquisition. Do an "out with the old" cleanup to make space for a fresh view on life.

A belief is a template of perception—it's the "norm" we come to automatically expect. Beliefs we assume to be "the absolute truth" are often shaped by:

1. Impressions made on our young minds by society, culture, parents, and leaders from our upbringing (aka other people's opinions that we've internalized)

2. Conclusions we made about ourselves and the world in order to cope from past negative experiences and trauma.

3. The ego wanting to protect itself so we look good and stay in our comfort zone.

Becoming conscious of your nonconscious, automatic beliefs gives you the ability to:

a) See the root of a belief—where it came from

b) Practice compassion toward yourself for however this belief became fixed

c) Soften and release the old belief so you can choose a *new* belief that is more empowering and true.

Sammie, a client who works in the film industry, said to me in one of our sessions, "I got the job of my dreams, but once I got it, I couldn't enjoy it because I was so worried about proving myself to everyone. I kept waiting for the other shoe to drop—feeling the fear and dread of the job ending."

The job eventually ended because it was a limited project working on a movie, and as she started applying for new jobs, she felt the fear creep in again. This time, her fear sounded like, "What if I haven't had enough experience and I'm not qualified enough to get another job in this field?"

I asked her, "But weren't you an executive producer for over two years on your last film?"

She said, "Yes!" And then took a deep breath. "Ya know what? I *am* qualified! I know I always do an excellent job whenever the opportunity presents itself."

"So," I asked, "what is the real fear?"

She thought about it and took another big breath. "Everything I do always has to be *so hard*. Getting the job is hard. Doing the job is hard. Losing the job is hard. Looking for a new job is hard."

I asked her, "How do you *want* to feel?"

"Fulfilled. I want to be happy with where I am. I want to have real faith and trust in the process."

"What's stopping you?" I asked.

"I believe that success always has to be hard for me—that I have to work my ass off to prove I'm worthy." We dove deeper into the core roots of this belief, and Sammie was able to find the connection between her parents' expectations for high achievement and how she continues to show up today in her work—always wanting to prove herself. She saw more clearly that now she wants to feel fulfilled internally on her own terms—regardless of external validation—but her pattern is to chase validation to prove she's worthy. Even once she gets the dream job, that's not enough because she quickly shifts into chasing the "I'm worthy" validation from bosses and superiors. So long as the belief is, *Validation and fulfillment are sourced on the outside of me,* her thoughts, strategies, feelings, and actions will be focused on getting a momentary hit of approval from an external source. Sammie's template of perception was entirely built around this belief: *It has to be hard for me.*

She attempted to tell herself things like, "Just trust," and "Have faith," and "Be patient," and "This is a part of your healing path," but in our session, she admitted that she knew she was saying the "right" affirmations to herself, but she wasn't yet believing these things—and trusting them to be true. I've been there. Before you splatter yourself with positive affirmations that sound like the "right thing" that you "should be" thinking, you must be willing to truthfully face and see the root of the belief. Then, you can understand where the belief is sourced from, locate its root, and give yourself the appropriate healing balm.

The mind seeks to affirm what it already believes to be true. The key to changing your template of perception is *to see* what's not working and *to question* what you've previously deemed unquestionable. The first step is to become aware of the belief that's got you stuck and isn't serving your True Self. Start by getting present to the negative thoughts—those autopilot beliefs that you just presume to be the absolute truth—and question their legitimacy. Here's a journal exercise for you to question—and get to the root of—a limiting belief:

1. *What is a limiting belief you hold about yourself—one that you know is keeping you stuck?*

2. *Thinking back as far as you can, where did this belief come from?*

3. *Is this belief helpful? Is it kind? Is it actually true?*

4. *What is the core desire within you that is seeking to be met? What do you really want or need?*

Understanding yourself in this deeper way, now invite your adult self to have compassion for the child version of yourself who has a core root need and longing that went—for whatever reason—unmet. For Sammie, her inner child's desire was to be acknowledged and seen. In order for her to *truly* have faith and trust, she needed to identify and consciously let go of the belief that *Everything needs to be hard* so she could experience her inherent self-worth.

Just as steaming your face before extracting a blackhead softens your skin, these questions help soften a hardened belief system that you once thought to be *absolutely fixed*. If a belief is unhelpful, unkind, and untrue, then it's taking up way more real estate in your mind than it's worth…it's a weed that is ready to be whacked! It's time to question the authenticity of these beliefs so you can flip the script and write a new narrative that illuminates your True Self. Let's look at how we can open the mind to see what is true instead of what is not.

DISSOLVE THE DELUSIONS

Twenty-twenty vision requires your willingness—and desire—to see through the bullshit. In the yoga tradition, *satya* means "truthfulness." The word *sat* means "that which exists, that which is." The essence of satya is seeing things as they actually are, not as we wish them to be. Your spiritual path asks that you not bypass the truth—but rather look at it with sober neutrality. Right now, this is *what is.*

The moment you deny *what is,* you turn on your back on an aspect of the truth. It takes courage and integrity and commitment to look at your life—and to keep it real with yourself. Satya allows you to pierce through the bullshit of noise and delusion and see the pure, potent, aliveness of the moment that you're in. You are willing to be courageous and deal with what is in front of you—not what you wish was, or wasn't, in front of you. Sometimes, we don't like what we see, so satya invites us to courageously see and face whatever shows up—including the tough stuff.

Pantanjali's *Yoga Sutras* identify this tough stuff as the five *kleshas,* or afflictions. "Klesha" is a term from Indian philosophy and yoga that means "poison." The five kleshas are the causes of all suffering—they cloud us from seeing the truth. Awareness of each of the kleshas can give you a way to dissolve the delusion and see your life through clear eyes.

Avidya: Ignorance

In Sanskrit, *vidya* means "knowledge," and so *avidya* is that which takes us away from knowledge—from remembering who we are. Avidya causes us to perceive the world through the lens of our individual, more superficial reality, perceptions, and goals—while believing that our perceptions are "right." This righteousness creates

a veil that hides the truth, which causes suffering because it's freaking painful to forget your innate wisdom. It's said that avidya is the
trunk of the tree and the other four kleshas are branches that emerge
from it.

Asmita: Egoism

Smita has multiple meanings including smiling, expanding, and
blossoming. *Asmita* is the opposite—not smiling, expanding, or blossoming. The ego is the sense of "I" or "me," which isn't inherently
wrong, but by becoming too self-obsessed and fixated on your own
personal gains without regard to your impact on others, you get rigidly
stuck and lose connection to the greater whole of life.

Raga: Attachment

Raga is attachment to pleasure—to the things we like. The suffering of raga is caused by preference for the good feelings that we get
from things like social media, sex, drugs, alcohol, coffee, chocolate,
validation, and the list goes on. Each one of these things can be won-
derfully awesome, but attachment causes a sense of loss, sadness, or
obsession when the desired experience comes to an inevitable end.

Dvesha: Aversion or Hatred

Dvesha is suffering caused by dislikes—the things you deem to be
"bad" or "wrong." It's often the push and pull between raga and
dvesha, attachment and aversion, likes and dislikes that causes suffering. This creates a judgment for the way life "should be" (a recipe for
misery) instead of acknowledging "what is" (the path of truth).

Abhinivesha: Fear of Death

Abhinivesha is the ultimate fear. Clinging to life creates a fear that causes you to obsess and worry about losing your life, instead of being fully in it now. Through the release of the clinging, you can be more fully in the moment now with a joyful and rich appreciation of life itself.

As you were reading, maybe you had an "Oh shit, that's me" moment. I always do! The kleshas take you away from knowing that you are connected to a Source that is much greater than what your five senses can perceive. By becoming conscious of where the kleshas arise in your life, you can get real with what might be holding you back from seeing the truth.

Now, imagine your vision is like the windshield of a car. At birth, your windshield is clean and clear. But as you move through life, shit happens. Dead bugs smash against it. A bird poops. More dead bugs. And it goes on. This shit on the windshield represents things like a tough breakup, a teacher who spoke to you in a condescending tone that made you want to give up, being bullied at lunch, feeling the impact of harming another person, regrets, losses, failures, successes, joys, all of it.

These life experiences create impressions that impact you on a deep level and inform how you see the world and experience yourself in it. In Sanskrit, these impressions are known as *samskaras*. Samskaras don't just live in the mental body. They land in all five koshas and make impressions on physical, energetic, subtle, and cellular levels.

Eventually, as you realize there's shit on your windshield, you turn on your windshield wipers to try and wash away the samskaras so you can see clearly, but it all just smears, and your vision gets even hazier. Eventually, this haziness becomes self-doubt. The thing is, on some level, you know you're not seeing clearly, so you begin to doubt yourself instead of realizing *There's gotta be a way to clean this thing!* So how can you clean the dirty windshield?

CLEAR EYES, FULL HEARTS, CAN'T LOSE

If samskaras are impressions that condition you to see the world through a limited lens, it is said that *practice* is the spoke in the wheel that interrupts this conditioning. Just as the afternoon sun burns the morning mist off of the shore of the ocean, spiritual practice is a discipline that lifts the veil of the optical delusion and purifies the dirty windshield. Spiritual practice can take the form of yoga, embodied movement, meditation, therapy, and many others. Transforming the mind to see satya, truthfulness, requires a daily, moment-to-moment practice of presence. The goal is to see yourself and the world around you with clear eyes—unfiltered by the disempowering stories and beliefs that have been handed down to you. Spiritual practice is the purification process that allows you to see with clear eyes and a full heart.

Just as you accumulate unconscious, shadowy samskaras, you can also plant conscious, healing samskaras that root, flower, and bloom from within. When I interviewed Harvard-trained neuroscientist and president of the Platypus Institute Dr. David Bach on "SoulFeed," he taught us how to rewire a neural pathway in the brain, which creates a new impression.

"First," he said, "you *interrupt* the pattern that is no longer desirable."

Then, "You *replace* the old pattern with a new one."

"*Repeat* this process until the new connection in your brain develops and deepens the groove of the new pattern in your mind."

Interrupt and replace. Repeat. Interrupt and replace. Repeat. Again and again until the new neural pathway is the new normal. Every time you *interrupt* an old pattern and *replace* it with a new one, you're not only strengthening your mental musculature—your mind's ability to form a new way of seeing—but you're *also* creating an impression that impacts all five koshas and begins to attune your nervous system to the truth. *This is how you shift gears and get on the path that you are meant to be on!*

Like any new habit, a new spiritual practice can be hardest at first, but it gets easier as the new neural pathway becomes the path of least resistance. For example, let's say you decide you want to start using your nondominant hand to brush your teeth. At first, this would feel weird and maybe even annoying. But since you're committed, each time you go to automatically use your dominant "normal" hand, you stop yourself in your tracks (interrupt) and then instead use your nondominant hand (replace). Using your nondominant hand will eventually become easy and natural with (repeated) practice. It may even eventually become the dominant hand. Success! While this is a pretty "low stakes" example, imagine the impact on your life when you apply this technique to what really matters to your soul.

This next practice is perhaps *the* most important exercise and practice of this book, on your journey to your truth. This practice is the "spoke in the wheel" of your life that creates a new and different way of living by intentionally creating a samskara that is in alignment with your True Self—one that is sourced from your wisdom, your soul, and your truth. Let's look at which samskaras are clouding your mind so you can choose to actively dissolve the delusion of an outdated narrative that is no longer serving you and the world.

SANKALPA: YOUR HIGHEST TRUTH

A *sankalpa* is a purified intention, without doubt. Translated literally from Sanskrit, *san* means "a connection with the highest truth," and *kapla* means "rule" or "vow." Your sankalpa is "the rule that follows the truth," as Tracee Stanley puts it. It is your commitment and resolve to be in alignment with your soul's highest truth.

Your sankalpa is more powerful than an intention because your sankalpa is sourced from your Wisdom body, your heart. An intention that is not purified comes from a place of doubt. For example, if someone fears not having enough money, they may say their intention is, "I want to save $10,000." That's a perfectly fine intention or goal; however, at the root, it's actually sourced from an energetic place of fear, lack, scarcity, and doubt. Like Sammie wanting the job.

You'll use language to articulate and spell out your sankalpa; however, the essence of your sankalpa is not sourced from a mental-cognitive place. It's sourced from deeper within you—from the truth of who you are. A sankalpa is different from your *why*, which is your dharma—your soul's purpose. Your sankalpa is a healing balm to a specific pattern that is not serving your True Self. You can have multiple sankalpas, but I tend to work with one for about six months to a year before moving onto a new one. A sankalpa is the vow you make to align with your *why* and get on your soul's true path.

I'm going to walk you through this process—inspired by the work of Rod Stryker and explained in his book *The Four Desires*—so you can purify self-doubt, tap into your truth, and make a vow that is sourced from a deep space of wisdom within. This sankalpa is your vow to make a conscious new impression within yourself that is in alignment with your highest truth—which influences the way you show up in the world.

As you answer the next questions, you'll receive clarity by getting down to the source roots of your disempowering belief:

1. *What are the three lessons you are tired of learning?* What are those recurring frustrations or repeated life patterns that keep coming up? *"Oh, not this again!"* Write one or two sentences for each lesson you are tired of learning.

2. *What is the story you are telling about yourself that keeps you stuck in this pattern and disconnects you from your True Self?* What does the story or narrative sound like? Write the words

on the page as an act of discharging and removing the strong-hold that this story has had on you. Let it out.

3. *What are you getting out of this story?* In other words, what is the payoff? There's always *something* you get out of the story/pattern. Can you identify what it is?

4. *From the three lessons you are tired of learning, what is the common theme?* Look at the three lessons and extract the commonality. The theme might sound something like, "I keep settling for less than I know I'm worth," or "I need to trust my gut." In Sammie's case, it was, "Everything has to be hard."

Okay, take a deep breath. You're almost there. It's time to write your sankalpa! Your sankalpa is not only a new narrative, but a new energetic intention and vow to allow the truth to unfold from within you and ripple out into your life. Here are some guidelines:

- Your sankalpa should be around one or two sentences. One sentence, if you can.

- Your sankalpa is written as the healing medicine, the balm to this common theme from the lessons you are tired of learning.

- Begin your sentence with "I can, I will, I must…" as directed by Swami Rama in his book *The Art of Joyful Living* (1989).

As an example, I'll share a sankalpa of mine so you can get a sense of what one might look like: "*I can, I will, I must…come out and express my bright, full, shining, badass self. I do this by singing, dancing, and filling every space I enter with voice, movement, and light.*" This sankapla came from a time in my life when I was hiding—when I felt undeserving of being seen and shining bright.

Write your sankalpa down somewhere that matters to you.

It's important to not only "think" about your sankalpa and repeat it in your mind, but also to embody and integrate it into both your conscious and subconscious space. So it can move into the five koshas and leave a lasting impression on your soul. Here are three invitations to integrate your sankalpa more deeply into your body and being:

1. Through the Yoga Nidra practice, you can "place" the vibration of your sankalpa into the sixty-one points of the body. This is a deeply relaxing practice that you're invited to do for forty days to receive the healing medicine of your sankalpa. Commit to this practice, and it will have a powerfully transformative impact on you and your life. I've recorded a forty-day Sankalpa Nidra meditation for you to do this practice at http://www.trustyourtruthbook.com.

2. Open your journal to two blank pages, side by side. Using magazines, photos, dried flowers, and more, identify images and items that resonate with your sankalpa. There is definitely no right or wrong here. Simply read your sankalpa and choose images and items that feel like a fully-body "Yes, that's it!" Paste these images and items on the two side-by-side pages. Place your open journal somewhere meaningful to you—somewhere you can see the images and be reminded of the essence, the vibration, of your truth.

3. Use your sankalpa to rewire the neural pathways in your brain. When an old belief arises, or a klesha clouds your vision, *interrupt* the pattern with awareness of what's happening. Then *replace* the thought with your sankapla. *Repeat* this throughout your days, wherever you are.

Your sankalpa has a vibration to it. It's your truth. The more that you practice bringing your conscious awareness to your sankalpa as a single point of focus, the more your truth is coming alive—from the inside out. Now let's move into what's possible when you surrender, trust, and let go.

CHAPTER 7

Surrender to Source

Crown Chakra, *Sahasrara*

Color: Violet

Element: No element (elementless)

Body: Top of the skull

Emotional Impact: Letting go of control and manipulating outcomes, surrendering to a Higher Power

Shadow: Attachment

Light: Divine connection

Soul Truth: *I surrender my soul to the Oneness of the Universe.*

Mantra: *Om* (Bringing the awareness to the space between the eyebrows, repeat om—sounds like "home"—out loud or silently eight times before beginning to read this chapter. After repeating, listen for the silence and sense the energy of spacious emptiness.)

It's time to remember who you *truly* are. Big picture. What's possible for your life when you remember your connection to Source, to Divine Power, to the Universe? In truth, the work of this chapter isn't much work at all. And yet, it can be the most challenging because trusting that we're supported and releasing the need to control outcomes can be where the most resistance comes up. For the part of you that may feel like you need to do it all alone—like you need to hold the weight of the world in your hands—I offer this to you.

Have you ever looked up at the stars at night and felt both big and small at the same time? That life is so much bigger than you, and yet, *you are life* itself? There's something so humbling, yet spiritually empowering, about the fact that we humans are a blip on the screen of the entire existence of the Universe. Here's a fun perspective: if the evolutionary timeline of the Universe from the Big Bang until now— *13.7 billion years*—was condensed into a calendar year (January through December), dinosaurs would reach their height at the top of the food chain on December 29, they would go extinct on December 30, and all of human existence thus far would happen on December 31. According to Carl Sagan's Cosmic Calendar from his book *The Dragons of Eden* (1977), we are currently living at 11:59 p.m. on December 31. When converted to this scale, each *second* represents 434 years!

So when you're hung up on the bills, the debt, the body, the noise, the doubt, the fear, the silliness…it can be helpful to remember that this brief life is YOURS. Fucking claim it. How would you breathe in this moment—this second—if you knew your breath was the equivalent of 434 years? You are living lifetimes—a continuation of the same Source energy that's been expanding and extending since the beginning of time.

Tapping into Truth, with a capital T, comes from connecting to Source—a power that is higher and greater than any single one of us. In Alcoholics Anonymous, they call this your Higher Power. You always have access to this Truth, but it can sometimes feel scary, or even impossible, to trust. When you are ready to let go of the heavy weights that are not yours to carry (and never were!), this is your invitation to trust in a power greater than you and be guided by the Source of life. To tap into your true power and embrace the magic, mystery, and magnitude of your life, READ ON, dear one! It's your time.

LOCATE YOUR HIGHER POWER

In my first interview with Caroline Myss, the beloved medical intuitive and author of *Anatomy of the Spirit,* she said, "Do you think the mind can get you to [connect with] God? It cannot! The mind's not your ally; it's your adversary because it wants proof all the time. Proof of what?! You think God's gonna show up or an angel's gonna show up or the room's gonna start rattling? If that happened, you'd wet your pants. When, in fact, God is everywhere in nature. It's in your nature. *Get back to your nature!*"

When you were young, there was likely a point when you were completely enamored with the mystery of life…full of wonder, awe, and curiosity. You were plugged into magical and unseen worlds, and your imagination was just as real—if not more real—than the "real world." The veil between you and Source was thinner because you weren't yet conditioned by the world's structures, narratives, and boxes. Its dos and don'ts. Shoulds and shouldn'ts. As adults, if we don't practice staying in communication with Source, we lose touch with the great mystery and become hardened by the world and attached to the kleshas—avoiding pain and attaching to pleasure, driven by our preferences.

Is there a word for Source that feels most appropriate for you? Divine, God, Goddess, All That Is, Higher Power, Universe, Energy, Consciousness.... What word or phrase do you feel called to name the great mysterious force of intelligence that somehow made it possible for you to be reading these words right now? From this point forward, you'll see me use different terms for Source to avoid getting fixed on any one "thing." By using different words, this energy may occur to you in a different way each time. Whenever you see a word that is my attempt to name this indescribable force, take a breath to notice what feels true *for you*. I'll also use "God-dess" to lift up that this all-encompassing energy includes both genders *and* the full spectrum of gender expression.

Growing up, I thought God was a man with a white beard in the sky. The God I had in my mind and knew my heart was never mean, judgmental, unkind, or angry. He was kinda like a Santa Clause type, a pretty chill dude! When I began to study and practice yoga, my understanding of God-dess deepened and widened to embrace a larger understanding. I share this with you—not to bestow upon you my own definition—but to encourage you to explore your own relationship with your Higher Power. Today, my understanding is that God-dess is *everything*. All of the things. And none of the things! Every particle of air, breeze of wind, every person, ant, bird, tree, and blade of grass. God-dess is within me and around me. God-dess is the oceans and the lakes, the rivers and the forests, the deserts and the mountains, the glaciers and the waterfalls. God-dess is present within every person, every smile, every breath, every mistake, every tragedy, every success, every win, every loss. Past and present. Human and being. Sun and moon. High and low. Man and woman and every being in between. God is everything and nothing. The Oneness from which all perceived "individuals" emerge.

Your relationship with Source is not only an energy outside of you; it's very much alive within you and may be experienced by you as your "inner truth." This relationship can be enlivened by connecting to the crown chakra, the top of your skull, which connects you to the unseen world beyond this physical "reality." It transcends the limitations of the material world. The Universe communicates to us through our five senses—touch, taste, smell, hearing, and sight—but is not limited to these senses alone. In fact, most of what's happening is undetectable by our senses, so we must stay open to the mystery! What are we *not* seeing?

Western culture has largely lost touch with the sacred. In our instant-gratification culture of social media and digital noise, creating time and space for stillness and quiet so you can cultivate a relationship with your Higher Power is becoming both increasingly rare and incredibly necessary. Let's do this embodied visualization meditation, as you read, to connect you with sahasrara, the crown chakra:

Bring your awareness to the top of your skull. Take a deep, full inhale in. Release a complete, cleansing exhale out.

As you inhale, sense that the breath is moving from the soles of the feet up to the crown of the head.

As you exhale, sense that the breath is moving from the crown of the head down to the soles of the feet.

Repeat this sweeping breath three times—from the soles of the feet to the crown of the head. From the crown of the head to the soles of the feet.

Now imagine there's a ring of healing light-energy floating six inches above the crown of the head.

Imagine this healing ring of light begins to emit streams of light downward—like rays of sun moving toward the top of the skull. Sense that the top of the skull is open and available to receive this stream of light—illuminating the center of the skull.

Feel this warm light energy move into the mind, and then the throat, the heart, the navel, the hips, and the legs—all the way down to the feet.

Sense that you are receiving divine life force energy through the crown of the head all the way down to the toes.

Notice your breath and bask in this light for a few moments, minutes, or as long as you wish.

MEANINGFUL SPIRITUAL PRACTICE

Imagine you're a child running barefoot through a field—feeling the cool dew beneath your glowing feet. You don't question your Oneness with all things. You are plugged-in—in playful flow with the Divine. As adults, we lose touch with this Oneness, so spiritual practice brings us back so we can remember. Sometimes we need to leave home to come home.

Spiritual practice is preparation—to get ready to connect to your Higher Power. It's the process of consciously transcending the societal conditioning that numbs you from this sacred force of Oneness. Like your sankalpa from chapter 6, it's the spoke in the wheel that allows you to overcome ignorance (avidya) and see the truth. *Any practice where you remember your connection to Source is a spiritual practice.* Crocheting; practicing yoga; meditation; prayer; taking a hike; AA; time in a church, synagogue, temple, or mosque; or standing under a waterfall. It can be done lying down or while running a marathon. It's less about the activity you are *doing* and more about the intention you're embodying with your *being.* Your willingness to give up the ego's agenda and devote yourself to a higher plan is the essence of the spiritual warrior. Any sacred space where you have an intention and willingness to give up the responsibility of having to manipulate, strategize, and "do it all yourself" is spiritual.

The word *spiritual*—broken down—is spirit-ritual. *Spirit* is the unseen aspect of your being—the Energy body, Mental body, Wisdom body, and Bliss body. *Ritual* is any sacred practice. Your commitment to developing your spiritual practice is a stake in the ground that says, "In a world that wants me to overidentify with the physical, material world, I refuse to forget who I am. I am committed to remembering my deep soul power."

SAY A LITTLE PRAYER FOR YOU

Source speaks to us in whispers and words, through inspired ideas, in waves of wind, in drizzles of rain, through the chirping of birds and voices of friends, and even the ringing of the phone. The question is not, "Is Source speaking to me?" The question is, "Am I listening?"

It is said that, "Prayer is asking. Meditation is listening." When you say a prayer, you are speaking directly to the deepest part of yourself *and* the whole Universe. A prayer can be as easy as asking a question. The prayer I say every day at the end of my yoga or meditation practice, hike, or workout is, *How may I be of service and share my gifts? Please show me the way.* Prayer is planting the seed of an intention. Meditation is creating space to make yourself available to hear the answers. *You must make the space.* Whenever I go on my favorite ninety-minute round trip hike from my home in Topanga Canyon, I make it a rule to leave my phone at home. I know if I don't consciously leave my phone behind, it'll eat up the space that I've dedicated to listening. The revelations I have as a result of this empty space are profound!

TAKE IT EASY

Recently, while I was doing some work I'd been procrastinating on, the internet went out. The worst! My first response was, "Are you fucking kidding me? NOW?! Of course this happens when I finally sit down to work on this!!" I could feel myself going to that place of "WHY ME?!" and feeling like a victim of this internet outage.

But instead of wasting energy, attempting to force the internet to work (a losing battle that always leads me to deeper frustration), I surrendered my personal agenda to my Higher Power's plan. I prayed, "How is this internet failure a part of the divine flow? Show me the way." My answer came quickly! As I surrendered the outcome, I got an email notification from the Apple store saying that my computer was repaired and ready for pick up several days early. *Score!* Instead of fighting with the internet a second longer, I embraced the especially beautiful day, rolled down the car windows, felt the warm wind blow on my skin, and put on "Take It Easy" by the Eagles. As I traversed down the canyon, I reminded myself of another sankalpa of mine, "It's safe to soften and surrender." And of course, as I walked into Apple, "Take It Easy" came on—playing through the whole store. Pure Divine Alignment (PDA). I knew I was in communication with a force greater than myself and through surrendering my personal agenda, I could experience life's plan, which always works out one way or another.... And hey! Sometimes, when you take it easy, it gets easier.

Cultivating your relationship with your Higher Power is a constant practice of presence, surrender, and trust. Feeling connected to this force is always one breath, one moment, one practice away. As we move forward in this chapter, I'll share practices that have profoundly helped me cultivate and enliven my relationship with God-dess. You'll also get a chance to inquire about some of the reasons why you might avoid this relationship at times—like so many of us do.

DEAL WITH DENIAL

Within you is God-dess-like potential—your innate ability to align with the highest Truth and be an expression of the Divine in human form. And yet, this human experience can feel so vulnerable and uncertain sometimes, you may struggle to trust you are supported. Faith is the practice of trust—without needing proof. They call it a *leap of faith* for a reason.

But, when you cling to quick fixes as a means to numb the tenderness and vulnerability, you end up getting hooked by the "fixes" and feel disconnected from the Divine. The ultimate cause of our suffering is our denial of connection to Source. This denial leads to an obsessive, often unconscious attempt to "fill the void." *We've all been there.*

When I interviewed Nikki Myers, the founder of Yoga of 12-Step Recovery (Y12SR) on "SoulFeed," she said, "Addiction is the disease of the lost self. I lose myself. And anytime I look outside of myself for something that can only come from the inside, I'm in a codependent relationship with whatever that thing is."

When we attempt to replace our Higher Power with someone or something material, we get addicted to the replacement. At the root of many people's addictions is a mistaken search for fulfillment in the material world and a need to numb the pain that comes from feeling disconnected from Source. Addiction is like plugging a lamp into a bag of Doritos and wondering why your lights won't turn on instead of plugging the lamp *into* the outlet itself. We think we'll get what we need…but we never do. Our addictive patterns sneakily make us believe we'll fill the void if we…

- Eat one more bag of chips

- Sleep with him one more time

- Take one more hit of the bowl

- Have one more cigarette

- Scroll through Instagram one more time

- Drink one more drink

- Insert your "one more" here.

Sometimes, I "write off" my own addictive patterns as "insignificant" and tell myself that, "Well, it's really not *that* bad," and "It's not like I'm doing _____ !" We try to make all kinds of things and people our "Source"—romantic partners, bosses, celebrities, cars, money, food, drugs, social media followers, sex.... But your relationship with all these things will suffer if you are looking to source your relationship with God-dess through them.

The addictive pattern I've struggled with the most is my relationship with my cell phone. The empty promise of the quick hit of dopamine—that "feel good" neurochemical that releases in my brain when I see more social media likes, follows, emails, and texts—distracts me from the empty space where I can access my connection with my Source. As I've tried to manage my relationship with my phone, I've wondered, *Why am I so scared of the empty space?* One reason is that I, like so many people today, have become accustomed to the constant stimulation and noise that comes from the smartphone. Another deeper reason is that I, like so many people today, am afraid to be alone with myself. To be in the stillness. The quiet. The void.

Scientists agree that the first human species emerged between five million and seven million years ago. And, guess what?! Smartphones became widespread around 2006! Needless to say, this type of constant, overwhelmingly nonstop noise and stimulation is quite new to the human species. Before the digital age, we spent way more time bored, alone with ourselves, and accessing our creative capacities. When we have empty space, our true creative potential can emerge. Out of the nothing comes the something.

> The areas of your life
> where you are most
> attached are the areas
> where the healing medicine
> of trust and faith are
> needed.
>
> ♡

In order to write this book that you're reading right now, I needed to turn my phone off for hours and even days at a time—so I could remove the noise and temptation to "binge scroll." Through my willingness to create a boundary and deal with this addictive pattern, I was able to access my Higher Power and cocreate the words and chapters of this book. In fact, most of the words you are reading were written by me, first, going into the deep Nidra state so I could tune into Source within myself.

Your greatest spiritual work is to reckon with the material attachments that are blocking your connection to Spirit. Where are you attached? How do you distract yourself from empty space? To be in conversation with your Higher Power, explore this for yourself. Usually the areas of your life where you are most attached, holding, gripping, clinging, controlling, and manipulating are the areas where the healing medicine of trust and faith are needed.

Here's the reckoning: When you are busily consuming the world's messaging, advertisements, and mental noise pollution, you are plugging into the world's agenda for you instead of your Higher Power's bigger plan. You can cultivate this relationship through prayer (intentionally *asking for guidance*) and meditation (willingly *listening for a clear answer*). Give it a try and notice what you discover.

LET GO AND BE HELD

When you believe that you, and you alone, are responsible for controlling yourself and the world, you erroneously try to play God-dess instead of cultivating a trusting relationship with your Higher Power. It's impossible to do it all yourself and hold the whole world in your hands. What if you're actually supported beyond your ability to comprehend?

The areas where we grip and hold on show us where we can practice letting go. And it's a practice. Notice your breath and ask yourself, *Is there an area of my life where I feel like I have to "be in total control" and "hold it all together"? Where I feel a fear-based "need" to control people, circumstances, and outcomes in my surroundings?* As you bring this to the light of your consciousness awareness, take a deep breath. Notice how you feel. Do you want to run and hide? Grab for something comfortable? Throw this book across the room? Notice any feelings, thoughts, or instant reactions that arise. As humans, we resist letting go and asking for support—often mistaking this for "weakness." We clench, tense up, and miss out on opportunities to be held by the Universe. You deserve to be supported, and great relief is possible when you let go.

Answer these five questions in your journal to practice letting go:

1. *Where in my life—right now or recently—am I attached to controlling the outcome and unwilling to let go?* This could be in any area of your life: with your parents, spouse, partner, children, colleagues at work, even an airplane's departure time. Look out for perfectionism.

2. *What is the underlying fear that is triggering my need to control?* Try to put the fear into a single statement, like "I'm afraid of being alone," or "I'm afraid I won't be able to pay my bills."

3. *Where do I feel the impact of gripping in my body?* We tend to hold and contract in certain places in our bodies when we're feeling the need to control. It could be a clenched fist, tense abdomen, or a nervous knee bouncing. Breathe and notice.

4. *What's the worst thing that could happen?* Take your fear to its end result if it were to come true. Think, *I'll die alone,* or *I'll miss my deadline and be a failure,* or *I'll be angry at myself for wasting so much time on my phone.* Instead of the fear being in the shadows, living as an undercurrent of tension, bring it to your conscious awareness.

5. *What might be possible if I were willing to let go of control in this area of my life?* Imagine this tension is a weight you are carrying like a backpack full of heavy bricks. What if you took this heavy weight off your back and put it down—even for a few moments? Imagine handing your backpack of bricks to your Higher Power. *Who could I be? What could I do? How could I feel if I could give this over to my Higher Power?*

If you experience resistance to the idea of surrendering, first of all—that's normal. Especially when you're new to exploring this relationship or when your past relationship with the idea of "God" has been informed by harmful dogma or misinterpretation. But consider this. It's through surrendering the need to control that you can come to know your greatest strength. Your True Self starts to come through.

THE SWEET ART OF SURRENDER

Like everything we've discussed in this book, surrender is not just an idea to think about. Surrender is an embodied practice of letting the nervous system rest into a state of deep peace. When the central nervous system shifts from the sympathetic (fight, flight, freeze, or faint) to the parasympathetic (rest and digest), the body can actually soften and become available to receive.

When you are tense with muscles clenched and a furrowed brow, it's more difficult for the Divine to communicate with and through you! It's like if you try to throw a quarter onto a big, bouncy rubber ball, the quarter will likely bounce right off and shoot in another direction. If you toss a quarter onto a California king-sized bed, the quarter will land softly and be received by the bed. Surrendering is an embodied practice of softening and letting go in all places and spaces in the body—so you can receive the intelligence of the Source within you.

The practice of Yoga Nidra invites us to come to a lying down position and to be held and received by the earth. In the practice, the Goddess Yoga Nidra, Mother Earth herself, holds you so you can completely let go into deep rest, as if you were being held in a cocoon of sweet support. Even right now as you read these words, as you inhale, notice if you can feel and sense the ground rising to support and hold the body. And, as you exhale, notice if you can feel and sense the body resting its weight down into the support of the ground.

At the end of chapter 6, I invited you to do a forty-day Yoga Nidra practice of "placing" your sankalpa as a vibration of light within the sixty-one points of the body. This is a transformative practice of letting go and surrendering. Reread your sankalpa and check in. Notice how it may provide a healing balm/invitation for you to trust and surrender into your Higher Power's support. Additionally, I recorded a Surrender to Source deep relaxation meditation practice for you to invite your nervous system and body to experience what it actually feels like to let go and be held. Go to http://www.trustyour truthbook.com to begin.

OPEN TO RECEIVE

When I was living in NYC, I once had a day off work where I took a hit of a joint and then exhaled into a luxurious bath. After a few deep breaths, I felt my nervous system relaxing and letting go, and then all of a sudden, a wave emotion came over me and I started sobbing. The wisdom of this emotion carried with it a very clear message, "Go see your Aunt Bonnie *as soon as possible.*" I knew she was sick with ovarian cancer and wasn't doing well, but I wasn't sure how close to the end it was. I immediately listened to this guidance, got on the phone with my dad, and started making plans. It took me exactly a week to get on a train to Philadelphia to see her, but I got there.

When I walked into her house and went up the stairs to see her in the hospice bed, I was surprised to see how frail she was. My cousin Ron let me know that she hadn't spoken since the night before and everyone had already said their good-byes. It was clear I'd arrived at the eleventh hour of her life. If you've ever been with someone who's close to passing, perhaps you know that palpable preciousness of life that you can feel in the room. *This room was vibrating.*

Her best friend Mrs. Cassidy said to me, "Shannon! Talk to her! She can hear you!" So I quickly started rolling through all my most favorite memories of us...miniature golf in the summers...the time she came to see me in *Oklahoma!* and was jumping up and down with pride and joy after the show. All of a sudden, she jolted. Her eyes shot open, and I thought, *Oh God! I just shocked my Aunt to death!* She yelled, "Shannon!" and grabbed my hand tightly as I continued to run through my most favorite memories. She quickly fell back asleep and after a while, the hand grip eventually released. I'd just made it. Late that night, she passed away.

The next day, my cousins told me that the last word she ever spoke was my name. This felt like an honor—and I took this as "passing of a torch," a reminder I'd always carry her spirit with me. For my Aunt Bonnie, God was another word for love, and she used this relationship to love people fully and unapologetically. If you walked into her house, she'd spin in circles and jump for joy. A few months prior to her passing, she shared with me, "You know, Shannon, if the Lord is ready for me, I'm ready to go. I've been to all my kids' weddings, and I've held most of my grandkids and watched them grow. If it's my time, I'm ready." Her faith in a power greater than herself allowed her to let go of her physical body with trust. I continue to be in awe of her willingness to let go and love big. Death is a potent teacher of how to live. It reminds us to seize this moment now, show up fully, do the damn thing, and love people without reservation. When we remember the preciousness of life, we can show up more fully in it.

A few years after my aunt passed, I took Seane Corn's class for the first time at a yoga festival. At the end of class, Seane was saying a prayer that was incredibly moving and resonating to the core of my being. Suddenly, I felt my skull tingle, then a wave of sensation moved through my spine, and then, I felt the essence of my Aunt Bonnie's presence at my back, as if I was being wrapped in her loving joy. I'd never had an experience like this before. It felt like a moment of divine grace and deep peace.

These experiences lift up three pivotal practices—which are essential as you cultivate *your relationship* with Source:

1. *Make yourself available.* Because I got stoned in that freaking bathtub, the incessant busyness of my life temporarily stopped. This made me more available to receive divine guidance. We don't necessarily need plant medicines to tap into our

connection to deep wisdom, but in that moment, that's what helped me open up to receive the message I needed to hear. When we let go, we open ourselves up to receive.

2. *Follow the inspiration.* The loud message I received came in the form of a wave of emotion. Not all the guidance I receive is so loud, but the key is, I listened, went with it, took action, and chose to let my heart lead me to my aunt in "divine timing." Synchronicity comes as a result of listening to the guidance you receive. When you follow the inspiration, you can flow with the current of life.

3. *Know you're where you're meant to be.* This moment now is the most divine moment of all time. The key to access Source is to fully *be here* in the potent now-ness of this moment. Whenever you embrace *this* moment as the most important one of your life, you wake up and can see, feel, and sense the signs that you are in divine flow—like when I felt my aunt at my back in Seane's class. What wisdom is trying to communicate with you—right now?

The greatest spiritual practice is learning to be in this moment now *and* to let it go as it passes away and turns into a new moment of now. You are gifted with this chance to be here in this body, on this planet, on this earth. As you journey forth, remember this: you are a gift, you are needed, and it's your time.

CHAPTER 8

Be the Whole You.
We Need You.

"A human being is a part of the whole called by us 'Universe,' a part limited in time and space. He experiences himself, his thoughts, and feelings as something separated from the rest—a kind of optical delusion of his consciousness. This delusion is a kind of prison for us, restricting us to our personal desires and to affection for a few persons nearest to us. Our task must be to free ourselves from this prison by widening our circle of compassion to embrace all living creatures and the whole of nature in its beauty."

—Albert Einstein

Something important is happening. You are becoming *you*. You've chosen the courageous path of being yourself, and every time you stand in your truth, take honest action, feel truth, speak truth, see truth, and connect to the Source of truth within, you become more YOU! *This is the true healing that's possible when you trust your truth.*

Your healing has an unimaginable impact that doesn't stop with you. When you heal, we *all* get free. Your healing ripples outward as an invitation for other people to heal and trust *their truths*. It ripples to influence your parents and their parents and their parents—through reckoning with intergenerational harm. It ripples forward into future generations to awaken the opportunity for new narratives. History and destiny converge in this moment now through the presence of YOU, and how you show up now...how you heal now, has a cosmic impact.

This moment on our planet is unlike any other in the history of humankind. We have more access to resources, information, communication, and each other than we've ever had before, and we're simultaneously reckoning with the traumatic wounding we've been holding in our personal and collective psyche for generations. The division we see in our world is nothing new; we're just finally waking up to it (and hopefully, our role in it). Whereas before, numbing kept us from feeling the depth of the wound, those same old tricks aren't working anymore because we're being called to wake up and feel— both on personal/individual levels *and* on societal/collective levels. It's as if more people than ever before are willing to see the truth.

Remember: There is no separation between what is happening "out there" and what's happening within you. What you see is not separate from you. It's time to reckon with and heal the disempowering narratives that were handed down to us by generations of patriarchy, racism, sexism, xenophobia, homophobia, white supremacy, ableism, genocide, war, and division. Now is not the time to turn our backs on the suffering of others, but to rise up and reckon! Because we're *all* inextricably connected, your energy has an unimaginable impact. And *you* get to choose who you want to be and how you show up in this life.

We *must* look at the disempowering narratives that we've consumed and understand that it's not our fault for consuming them, but it is our responsibility to rewrite them. And we must look at how our own actions may perpetuate unconscious harm and suffering onto others. After all, a culture that says that any single one of us is less than worthy is not a culture grounded in truth. By owning your own sovereign divinity and true nature, you awaken to the divinity of *all beings*.

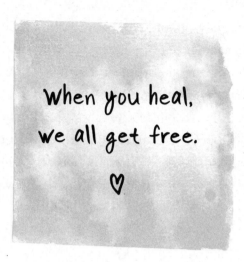

When you heal,
we all get free.

♡

The true source of self-doubt is unconsciousness. And what we're unconscious of is our innate power and inextricable connection to one another. So, whenever you remember your connection to Source and your responsibility to your fellow soul siblings on this planet, you return home to your true, conscious power. Self-doubt dissolves in the presence of Oneness.

We need *you* now. It's time.

You are the manifestation of God-dess-like power—of incredible potency, presence, wonder, and awe-inspiring magnificence. It's your time to claim your right to have freedom, power, and choice over your own energy field—your body, truth, and life. This moment is *yours*—an invitation to reclaim your power and live your badass life.

We need you, you matter, and you are powerful beyond measure. Your power is a permission slip to everyone around you to prioritize their healing and to step into their power, too. So, be the lighthouse! Be the light. Be the one who lights the way and inspires other people to see, know, claim, and reckon with their own shadow *and* light.

This journey is not guaranteed to be easy, but it is guaranteed to be yours. *So long as you claim it.* So, step into your truth, wake up, become conscious, see clearly, speak truthfully, love wholeheartedly, take action, create what you were born to create, and stand in the values of who you are here to be. Let people's jaws drop when YOUR badass walks into the room. Let them yearn to find that level of confidence and power within themselves too.

And, when they ask you if you've "always been so freaking fierce," look them straight in the eyes and tell them the truth of your journey. Show them your lows as well your highs. Support them to remember that they, too, can journey home to trust themselves—*that it's a practice.*

It's time to illuminate the *whole* of who you are—*all* of the colors of you—from the crown of your head to the soles of your feet. What is possible when you embrace *all* of you? When you let all of your true colors shine and taste the rainbow of your own magic? What does it look like to be the whole you—the complex you, the messy you, the contradictory you, the paradoxical you? In order for our world to heal, we need the whole you! So, let's invite ALL of you to have a seat at the table of your badass life. *Visualize with me.*

Imagine the earthen, red roots of your legs and the base of your spine—the root chakra—grounding you into this moment and reminding you that you belong here.

Imagine the color orange in your hips and pelvis, the possibility of your creativity and sexuality—the sacral chakra—inviting you to flow and dance and create your unique gifts for the world.

Imagine a bright yellow sun at the center of your navel, your connection to your sense of self and confidence—the solar plexus chakra—fueling the fire of your ability to courageously take action and feel your true power.

Imagine green, fresh new life blossoming in the center of your chest, your connection to your emotional power center—the heart chakra—empowering you to feel and express yourself truly.

Imagine crystal clear blue waves of air vibrating at the center of your throat, your connection to your voice—the throat chakra—inspiring you to speak truth that is in alignment with the vibration of your soul.

Imagine your mind illuminating with the color indigo, your ability to see the truth and yourself clearly—the third eye chakra—inviting you to see from a higher mind of intuitive perception.

Imagine a violet light glowing at the top of your head, your connection to the knowing that this is so much bigger than you—the crown chakra—plugging you into a Higher Power that allows you to connect to the true Source of who you are.

Know that each wheel of energy within you is your truth radiating and vibrating. It's circling and creating an energetic vibration that you carry with you in every space that you enter, in every moment of your life. Your work, my friend, is to allow the colors of your inner rainbow to shine fucking bright. To be all that you are capable of being. Your energy field is spinning with light, from head to toe, from back to front, from deep inside of you, and all around you. YOU are the one that we are waiting for.

So, get wild! Be the whole of who you are. Trust the journey. Trust the path. Trust yourself. And trust your truth because you deserve to be here and we need you now.

Imagine a world in which we ALL know how to honor ourselves and one another, embrace both the shadow and the light, and let no aspect of ourselves go unloved.

This is the transformative power of trusting yourself and encouraging other people to do the same. Self-doubt will arise, as it does, but the biggest difference you'll notice as you keep trusting your truth is: *you simply won't believe that voice.* A newer and truer voice—the voice of your soul—will emerge from the depths of your being to remind you of who you truly are.

Congratulations. You're the one you've been waiting for. You are worthy of not only living your badass life, but of being in deep alignment with your soul's purpose. Thank you, from the bottom of my heart for being on this journey with me. Thank you for having the courage to love yourself wholeheartedly and the willingness to trust your truth—down to your bones.

This is how we heal ourselves and transform our world. It starts with you, it ripples outward, and it always comes back around. May you take everything you've learned about yourself from the work you've done in this book and allow it to inspire you into confident action that continues to heal yourself and the world. It's time to live your badass life. *So be it. And so it is.*

Love,

Shannon

P.S. The Be the Whole You meditation practice as well as the full album of Trust Your Truth meditation practices for each chapter/chakra can be downloaded at http://www.trustyourtruthbook.com.

Acknowledgments

Words cannot express my gratitude for the many people who helped bring this book to life. First and foremost, thank you to New Harbinger for trusting me to write a book and making me an author—especially to Elizabeth Hollis Hansen, who believed in me from day one, Jennifer Holder for your wisdom and guidance, and my copyeditor Gretel Hakanson for your skillful eye and encouragement.

Thank you to Lindsay Samakow and Megan Monahan for pushing and convincing me to write a book before I was "ready."

Thank you to my dear friend, editor, and writing coach Jennifer Howd (http://www.jenniferhowd.com) for helping me shape the proposal for this book. Your attention, love, and guidance were essential as I built confidence in my writing process. This book would not exist without you.

Thank you to my dear friend and web designer Brea Galper (http://www.stylestoryteller.com) for your love, passion, creativity, and whole-hearted contribution to the web page for this book.

Thank you to Justin Michael Williams, my soul sibling, for cheering me through this whole process from the very beginning. I love you!

Thank you to my sweet, tenacious agent Gareth Esersky from the Carol Mann Agency who made sure *Trust Your Truth* found its perfect home.

Thank you to Laurén Jones and Jason Beekman for your invaluable feedback on the manuscript.

I couldn't have written this book without the essential support of my therapists Ciuin Doherty and Debbie Schiffman. Thank you for helping me process much of the healing I was able to share in this book.

Thank you Rupa Mehta for plucking me out from behind the front desk of my job at a yoga studio on the Upper West Side and making sure I did the Nalini Method teacher training. Your belief in me propelled me into my work as a teacher.

Thank you to my "SoulFeed" co-creator Alex Kip for pushing us to get to work and put something meaningful out into the world. Without your fire, I would not be standing where I am today.

Thank you to my sister Molly for being my soul sister and best friend. Your ability to understand me and validate my feelings (while always making me laugh!) is the greatest gift.

Thank you to my students and clients. You are my heroes! I'll never take for granted that you trust me to be a supportive guide for you on your path. Your courage and willingness to show up inspires me to keep going.

Thank you to Cindy Fukui Gim—your love, friendship, and warm welcome into your home has been one of the greatest gifts I've ever received. I wish the whole world could be like you!

Thank you to the Spitulnik Family for all the shabbat dinners, laughter, and for always making me feel home in your company.

Thank you to all my friends—my cheerleaders and my rocks. You know who you are. *I love you all so much.*

Thank you to Lauren Taus for showing me what unconditional love and friendship looks like. Thank you to all the powerful women in my life—especially Shannon Tyo, Florrie Bagel, Alexa Silvaggio, Kerri Kelly, and Naada Guerra.

Thank you to my entire family—my incredible parents Michael and Susan and the whole Algeo clan. And to my sweet, incredible brother Patrick for encouraging me, being proud of me, and inspiring some of this book. I love you, Patty.

MORE BOOKS

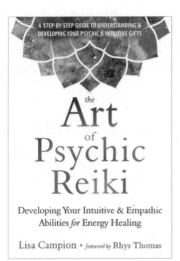

ISBN: 978-1684031214 | US $19.95

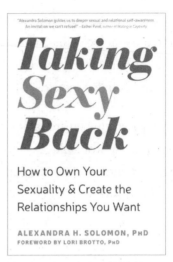

ISBN: 978-1684033461 | US $17.95

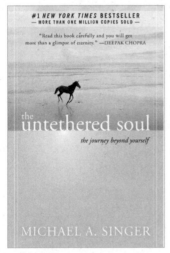

ISBN: 978-1572245372 | US $18.95

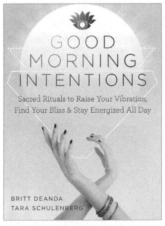

ISBN: 978-1-84035724 | US $18.95

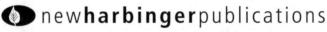

newharbingerpublications

NON-DUALITY PRESS | REVEAL PRESS

Named one of the "35 Under 35 in Wellness to Watch" by Wanderlust, **Shannon Algeo** is a celebrated speaker, writer, life coach, and Yoga Nidra and meditation teacher. His popular podcast, *SoulFeed*, features interviews with iconic cultural and spiritual leaders like Deepak Chopra, Caroline Myss, Marianne Williamson, Danielle LaPorte, and many more. In his coaching practice, Algeo works with clients to heal old patterns of trauma so they can show up in the world with power, presence, and purpose.

Algeo is known around the world for his gift of processing his own life experience into words that can be heard or read in service of greater learning, deeper resonance, and profound healing.

Algeo was rated as one of the "nicest instructors in New York City" by RateYourBurn for his work as a yoga and meditation teacher, and he leads meditation programs for companies like the global non-profit, (RED), founded by Bono and The Museum of Contemporary Art. In addition to giving presentations for Lululemon and the Wanderlust Festival, Algeo was a featured guest speaker at the United Nations "Yoga and the UN Culture of Peace" event. He is currently pursuing an MA in counseling psychology from Pacifica Graduate Institute.

Register your **new harbinger** titles for additional benefits!

When you register your **new harbinger** title—purchased in any format, from any source—you get access to benefits like the following:

- Downloadable accessories like printable worksheets and extra content
- Instructional videos and audio files
- Information about updates, corrections, and new editions

Not every title has accessories, but we're adding new material all the time.

Access free accessories in 3 easy steps:

1. Sign in at NewHarbinger.com (or **register** to create an account).

2. Click on **register a book**. Search for your title and click the **register** button when it appears.

3. Click on the **book cover or title** to go to its details page. Click on **accessories** to view and access files.

That's all there is to it!

If you need help, visit:

NewHarbinger.com/accessories

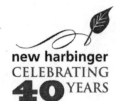

new harbinger
CELEBRATING
40 YEARS